Praise for *The Council of Dads*

"Reading *The Council of Dads* . . . remind[s] us which values we value most, and help[s] us make sure we transmit them." —*Time*

"Candid and moving. *The Council of Dads* exemplifies the mysterious process by which bad news can alter our perspective and reorder our priorities, and it celebrates the ever-expanding level of emotional intimacy that men are increasingly free to engage." —*Washington Post*

"Inspiring. . . . Changed the lives of everyone involved. . . . Ladies, there's no reason you can't start a council of moms. Let's just say every parent of a teenager could use some help and support!" —*Oprah.com*

"An incredible story and amazing idea." —Lance Armstrong

"Intimate." —*New York Times Book Review*

"Thoughtful. . . . From other men close to him, Feiler gleaned the qualities of curiosity and the urge to travel and learn, of taking care of things and people that matter, of remembering those who matter and casting them in a positive light." —*St. Louis Post-Dispatch*

D0973124

"As a doctor, I watch people facing death daily. As a reporter, I have gone to dangerous places and have often been put in harm's way. As a father of three girls I have often thought, 'What if something happens to me?' It is a frightening prospect and a daunting question. Recently I met a man who had a remarkable answer to that question. The story of Bruce Feiler profoundly connected with me and left me speechless. It made me rethink how I'd live my life and how I would take care of the three little girls I might leave behind."   —Sanjay Gupta, CNN.com

"Moving."   —*New York Daily News*

"Feiler tackles personal hardship with inquisitive and heartfelt eloquence."   —*Kirkus Reviews*

"A book that will touch many."   —*Booklist*

"Stirring. . . . A heartfelt meditation on parenthood, masculinity, and living life to its fullest. . . . Portraits of Feiler's own father figures and his council of dads [are] honest, heartfelt, and exceedingly raw. The book's power comes in part from Feiler's willingness to delve into emotions—including feelings of tenderness not only for our children and spouses but between male friends—that aren't often spoken of with such candor."   —*Hemispheres*

"It's hard not to get swept along and cheer Feiler on as he fights for his life and his daughters."
                    —*Publishers Weekly* (starred review)

"An uplifting lesson in parenthood."
—*The Daily Telegraph* (UK)

"Wonderful." —*Savannah Morning News*

"Feiler's council brings us all closer."
—*The Sun-Herald* (Sydney, Australia)

"A thoughtful, candid story of how the humdrum of everyday life can suddenly give way to upheaval, and of coming face to face with mortality. . . . A triumph."
—*The Age* (Melbourne, Australia)

"Bruce Feiler's unique approach to his cancer fight will get you thinking about family and the preciousness of life." —Livestrong blog

"Incredible." —*Daily Mirror* (UK)

"Feiler writes eloquently of his medical struggles and the exceptional men who stood by him and his family."
—*Oak Ridger* (Oak Ridge, Tennessee)

"Beautiful. . . . This book is very thought provoking."
—*Daily Mercury* (Mackay, Australia)

THE COUNCIL OF DADS

ALSO BY BRUCE FEILER

America's Prophet
Moses and the American Story

Where God Was Born
A Daring Adventure Through the Bible's Greatest Stories

Abraham
A Journey to the Heart of Three Faiths

Walking the Bible
A Journey by Land Through the Five Books of Moses

Dreaming Out Loud
*Garth Brooks, Wynonna Judd, Wade Hayes, and the
Changing Face of Nashville*

Under the Big Top
A Season with the Circus

Looking for Class
Days and Nights at Oxford and Cambridge

Learning to Bow
Inside the Heart of Japan

Walking the Bible
A Photographic Journey

Walking the Bible
*An Illustrated Journey for Kids Through the Greatest
Stories Ever Told*

THE COUNCIL OF DADS

A Story of Family, Friendship
& Learning How to Live

BRUCE FEILER

HARPER PERENNIAL

NEW YORK • LONDON • TORONTO • SYDNEY • NEW DELHI • AUCKLAND

HARPER ⬤ PERENNIAL

Photograph on p. vii by Edwin Feiler; photograph on p. 235 by Kelly Hike.

A hardcover edition of this book was published in 2010 by William Morrow, an imprint of HarperCollins Publishers.

THE COUNCIL OF DADS. Copyright © 2010 by Bruce Feiler. All rights reserved. Printed in the United States of America. No part of this book may be used or reproduced in any manner whatsoever without written permission except in the case of brief quotations embodied in critical articles and reviews. For information address HarperCollins Publishers, 10 East 53rd Street, New York, NY 10022.

HarperCollins books may be purchased for educational, business, or sales promotional use. For information please write: Special Markets Department, HarperCollins Publishers, 10 East 53rd Street, New York, NY 10022.

FIRST HARPER PERENNIAL EDITION PUBLISHED 2011.

The Library of Congress has catalogued the hardcover edition as follows:

Feiler, Bruce S.
    The council of dads : my daughters, my illness, and the men who could be me / Bruce Feiler. — 1st ed.
        p. cm.
    ISBN 978-0-06-177876-6
    1. Feiler, Bruce S.—Health. 2. Bones—Cancer—Patients—New York—Biography. 3. Father figures. 4. Children of cancer patients. I. Title.
RC280.B6F45 2010
362.196'994710092—dc22
[B]
                                                        2009041487

ISBN 978-0-06-177877-3 (pbk.)

11 12 13 14 15 OV/RRD 10 9 8 7 6 5 4 3 2 1

For my father
Keep walking

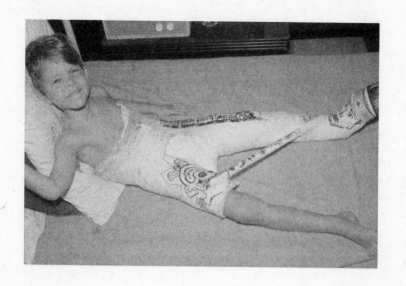

CONTENTS

x Contents

Time present and time past
Are both perhaps present in time future.

THE COUNCIL OF DADS

THE ORANGE STING-RAY

THE BIKE WAS BRIGHT ORANGE. It was a Schwinn Sting-Ray with a swooping banana seat, a miniature front wheel, and handlebars called "ape-hangers" because the grips rose so high they made the rider look like an orangutan. Modeled after hot rod motorcycles, the Sting-Ray was the most popular bike in America in the spring of 1970. My parents had given me one for my fifth birthday a few months earlier, and it was my most prized possession.

One day it almost cost me my life.

My family had recently moved to the south side of Savannah, Georgia, into a neighborhood where all the streets were named after Confederate generals—Johnston, McLaws, Early, Stuart. The idea that a century after the Civil War, socially conscious Savannahians would flock to a subdivision that memorialized the Lost Cause was a mark of how proud many Southerners still were at the tail end of the civil rights movement. We lived at 330 Lee Boulevard in a contemporary stucco ranch house built by my parents.

Late one afternoon I was exploring the neighborhood with my friend Scotty Sutlive when we came upon Pickett Circle, a small, magnolia-lined appendage off nearby Johnston Street that none of the other streets seemed to have. A secret discovery! We must return for more reconnaissance!

Racing home along the shoulder of Habersham Street, a heavily trafficked, two-lane thoroughfare that bisected our neighborhood, I had a brilliant thought. Why waste precious seconds turning around in Lee Boulevard? I could make a hasty 180 on Habersham and be back at Pickett Circle in no time. As Scotty lamely pedaled into Lee Boulevard (Hah! You'll never be a spy!), I deftly veered my bike into Habersham and was promptly—screech!—smashed by an oncoming sedan.

Wham.

My mangled Sting-Ray flew in one direction. My lacerated body in another. For a second I just lay in the road, my body stretched across the yellow line, feeling the warm pavement underneath my head. The owner of the house on the corner, Polly Meddin, suddenly appeared from her garage and came sprinting to my side.

Her shadow crossed my face. "Andy! Andy!" she cried, using my older brother's name. "Are you okay?"

"I'm Bruce," I replied, and promptly passed out.

———

I WOKE UP THE next morning in the hospital, unable to move. A plaster body cast stretched from my chest to my left toes, then down the opposite leg to my right knee. A steel bar ran from my right knee to my left foot. I had broken my left femur, the largest bone in my body. For the next two months I would lie flat on my back.

Back at home, my parents set me up in my bedroom, with a large folding table nearby, where I could pile all the toys I was getting. On top was a replica of the Apollo 11 command module that had splashed into the Pacific a year earlier. My mother, a junior high school art teacher, wanted to paint my cast, but I wouldn't let her until the day before it was scheduled to come off. We held our Passover seder in my room that year, and when the time came to hide the *afikomen* matzah—the highlight for young children, who receive a prize for discovering it—my father asked me to close my eyes and lift my head. He hid the treasure underneath my pillow.

For the next thirty-eight years, my broken left femur was the only medically interesting thing that ever happened to me. When I would visit a new doctor, I had only a few words to pencil in as I raced through page after page of ailments on the medical history forms. The truth was, I no longer thought about my broken leg. The only time it affected me was when I tried on shoes, since my recovery corresponded with a growth spurt, leaving my left foot a half-size larger than my right. But overall I was healthy. I looked younger than my age. I almost never saw a doctor.

And, on top of it all, I made a living by walking. For more than two decades I traveled the world and wrote about my experiences walking in other people's shoes. I taught junior high school in rural Japan; I earned a graduate degree in England; I performed as a clown under a traveling American big top; I crisscrossed the United States with Garth Brooks and other Nashville stars. And for the last ten years I had retraced the Bible through the war zones of the Middle East—climbing Mount Ararat in Turkey, crossing the Red Sea in Egypt, spelunking in caves in Jerusalem, airlifting into Baghdad, trekking across Iran.

Walking the Bible became a bestseller; the television series of the same name was seen around the world. I was the "walking" guy. The tag had become so indelible—and so aligned with my desire to be an experientialist—that on the last Thursday in June, thirty-eight years after my accident, I had dinner with my publisher and proposed an idea: I would spend the next ten years retracing the journeys of American history. I would follow its paths.

I would walk America.

We toasted the idea. I went home to bed. But the next morning, unbeknownst to anyone other than my wife, I went to the nuclear medicine department at New York–Presbyterian Hospital on Manhattan's Upper East Side to get what's known as a full-body bone scan. I had been directed to do this by a doctor I barely knew. A year earlier, our beloved family physician announced she was leaving our insurance plan, and I arranged for a farewell physical. All clear. For ten months I didn't see a doctor, which was normal for me. Finally, in May, I got around to finding a new internist, who ordered some routine blood work in our introductory meeting.

The next day she called. My alkaline phosphatase number was a little high, she said. 235. I didn't know what to think of this, because I had never heard the term. Alk phos, the doctor explained, is an enzyme in the blood that flags issues related to the liver or bones. She speculated that my level was probably high naturally, but she wondered if I'd had it tested before. A quick call to my previous physician revealed that I had, and that my alk phos number the previous July had been 90, perfectly normal. "Hmmm," my new doctor said. "That's surprising. Why don't we test it again? It's probably just a lab error."

It wasn't. The subsequent test produced a similar elevated number, and an additional exam ruled out any problems in my liver. That left my bones. She didn't think I had Paget's disease, an ailment common in older people whose bones and/or joints are beginning to deteriorate. On what sounded like a whim, she suggested I get a full-body bone scan. "Again, just to be sure," she said. "I'm sure it's nothing."

The Department of Nuclear Medicine is located on the second floor of New York Hospital. I was ushered into a crowded hallway and seated in front of a rolling table. A nurse stuck a needle into a vein in the back of my hand and injected what seemed like a Three Mile Island amount of radioactive tracers directly into my bloodstream. The sensation was chilling; I tasted a metallic backwash in my mouth. I was sent away for three hours and told to drink a lot and pee often.

After lunch I was led into a large room filled with what looked like a giant, robotic daddy longlegs. Stripped of anything metallic, I was strapped to a narrow bench and wrapped in a blanket while the snout of the machine, a huge metal plate, was lowered to an inch and a half above my nose. A bone scan is basically the opposite of an X-ray. An X-ray projects radiation into your body and uses it to create an image; a bone scan draws out the radiation that has been injected into your body and uses it to create the image. An X-ray takes less than a second; a bone scan lasts longer than an hour.

I was about thirty-five minutes into my scan, with the machine over my legs, when the technician suddenly popped out of his cockpit. "Did you have an accident involving your left leg recently?" he asked. I gulped. "I broke that femur when I was five," I said, hopeful. He nodded, disappeared into the hall, and for the next twenty minutes proceeded to talk very animatedly with the other technicians, just outside the door, all within plain sight. Two technicians then rescanned my leg from several angles but refused to answer my increasingly anxious entreaties about what they might have seen. "You have to talk with the doctors tomorrow," they said.

Tomorrow was Saturday, and there was no doctor to talk to me. By the time Monday rolled around—two centuries later—I could barely function, but again my doctor seemed unconcerned. "It's not like you have cancer," she said. "But still," she continued, "I've never seen anything like this. I think you should get an X-ray." On Tuesday, after she examined the X-ray, her tone had shifted. "You have an abnormal growth in your leg," she declared.

"You mean a tumor?"

"All abnormal growths are tumors," she said. "That doesn't necessarily mean anything."

But she ordered an MRI, and this time I didn't wait around for the official reading. I couriered the films a few blocks away to a family friend, Beth, who's an orthopedist. I paced York Avenue. Beth called just as the late-afternoon sun was shimmering off the surface of the East River. "I've looked at your scans," she said. "I insisted the top radiologist in the hospital do the same. And we both agree." Here she paused to choose the right language. "The growth in your leg is not consistent with a benign tumor."

I stopped walking. For a second I waited for the

double negative to convert itself into a single, much more devastating negative. *Not consistent with a benign tumor* could mean only one thing. She waited for me to complete the thought.

"I have cancer."

Then Beth was talking, and I was no longer listening. I needed to come to her office to get crutches. I needed to see this special surgeon she knew. I needed to call my wife.

I couldn't move. I sat down on a stoop. It was just like that moment, nearly four decades earlier, when I lay on the warm pavement of Habersham Street, knowing I had just been hit by the hardest force I could imagine, but not knowing what was going to happen next. And to think the tumor was in the same leg, the same bone, the same spot in my body. It couldn't be a coincidence. One thing, however, I already knew. I had spent my life dreaming, traveling, and walking.

Now I might never walk again.

2

THE COUNCIL OF DADS

Dear —,

As you know, I have learned that I have a seven-inch cancerous tumor in my left femur. The afternoon I first heard the diagnosis I was standing on York Avenue in Manhattan. I sat on a stoop, telephoned Linda, called my parents, and wept. I went to get some crutches, stumbled home, lay down on my bed, and stared at the sky for several hours imagining all the ways my life would change.

Then Eden and Tybee came in, running and giggling and looking in the mirror. They began to do this dance they made up when they turned three a few months ago. Mixing ring-around-the-rosy, ballet, and the hokey pokey, they twirled frantically in a circle, going faster and faster until they tumbled onto the ground, laughing with all the glee in the world. As I watched them, I couldn't control myself. I crumbled. I kept imagining all the walks I might not take with them, the ballet recitals I might not see, the art projects I might not mess up, the boyfriends I might not scowl at, the aisles I might not walk down.

The next few days were a tangle of tears and late-night conversations, doctor consultations, insurance negotiations, determination, hopes, and fears. I quickly determined I was looking at one of three options: the lost year, the lost limb, or the lost life.

Through it all, I kept thinking I would be fine. Whatever happens, I have lived a full life. I have traveled the world. I have written ten books. I am at peace.

I also thought Linda would be fine. She would experience a lot of pain and inconvenience, but in the end she would find a way to live a life of passion and joy.

But I kept coming back to Eden and Tybee and how difficult life might be for them. Would they wonder who I was? Would they wonder what I thought? Would they yearn for my approval, my discipline, my love?

My voice.

A few days later, I woke up suddenly before dawn and thought of a way I might help re-create my voice for them. I started making a list of six men—from all parts of my life, beginning with when I was a child and stretching through today. These are the men who know me best. The men who share my values. The men who helped shape and guide me. The men who traveled with me, studied with me, have been through pain and happiness with me.

Men who know my voice.

That morning I began composing this letter.

I believe my daughters will have plenty of resources in their lives. They'll have loving families. They'll have welcoming homes. They'll have each other. But they may not have me. They may not have their dad.

Will you help be their dad?

Will you listen in on them? Will you answer their questions? Will you take them out to lunch every now and then? Will you go to a soccer game if you're in town? Will you watch their ballet moves for the umpteenth time? When they get older, will you indulge them in a new pair of shoes? Or buy them a new cell phone, or some other gadget I can't even imagine right now? Will you give them advice? Will you be tough as I would be? Will you help them out in a crisis? And as time passes, will you invite them to a family gathering on occasion? Will you introduce them to somebody who might help one of their dreams come true? Will you tell them what I would be thinking? Will you tell them how proud I would be?

Will you be my voice?

And as I lay on my bed that morning, hoping I didn't wake Linda as I shook with tears, I said to myself that I would call this group of men "The Council of Dads."

The Council of Dads. Six men. All very busy and burdened with their own challenges, but together, collectively, they might help father my potentially fatherless daughters.

Naturally I hope that I will fully recover from my illness and that we will all be able to enjoy many family occasions together in the future. But I would like my Council to continue no matter the outcome. I would like my daughters to know the world through all of you. I would like Tybee and Eden to know me through this group.

I would like them to know themselves through their Council of Dads.

I understand this request might come as something of a burden. It is not intended to be an overwhelming commitment of time, resources, or emotion. A few words, a few gestures, an open door, a welcome embrace every now and then will ensure that your presence will be a constant guide in the girls' lives.

Your voice will merge with mine.

Even though it has been painful to write—and to contemplate—this unexpected idea at this moment in our lives has brought great strength and comfort to Linda and me. We are pleased to know that our girls will learn from you some of the valuable lessons you have taught me over the years. We are thrilled that we all have an excuse to keep more closely in touch in the seasons to come. And we are honored to add your fatherly counsel into the heart of our family.

And above all, we know that this assembly of surrogate dads can, if needed, be me.

Love,

Bruce

3

TWENTY FINGERS
AND TWENTY TOES

LIKE MANY YOUNG COUPLES, WE talked about having children. We dreamed. We feared. We picked out names. And we occasionally rolled our eyes at our mothers, who probed—not so subtly—about whether we had, er, news? One night my father-in-law, Alan, an attorney and elder sage around Boston, called rather late. No doubt his wife and high school sweetheart, Debbie, concerned that her thirty-something daughter had waited too late to get pregnant, was making one of her nightly trips to the Internet to hunt for frozen eggs or surrogate wombs, even though we had no reason to suspect we needed such things. "Are you busy?" Alan asked, more hopeful than concerned.

"Hey, Linda!" I called. "Your father wants to know if we're having sex."

"Are you kidding?" Alan responded. "If you promise not to use protection, Debbie will come over and light the candles!"

The truth is, we had made a schedule. Linda and I had met six years earlier on a blind date outside a gourmet food market on Twenty-third Street in Manhattan. She was wearing long flowing black silk pants and black patent leather high-heeled clogs, and her hair cascaded around her olive-skinned face like Sophia Loren's. With wide, chocolate brown eyes and a beaming white smile she could have passed for Latin, Italian, or Tahitian. She was my passport come to life.

But she had grown up in suburban Boston in a tight-knit family with a station wagon, a favorite pot roast recipe, and a nightly habit of eating ice cream out of coffee mugs standing alongside an open freezer. In other words, she was just like me. She loved to travel. She had recently started an international nonprofit called Endeavor that supported young entrepreneurs in the developing world. But she also loved to be home—to play Scrabble, do the Sunday crossword, and lament the scourge of green food coloring in mint chocolate chip ice cream.

We were engaged four years later on a balcony overlooking the Atlantic, and the next day Linda stunned me by announcing she wanted to get married in Savannah. "You come from a place of such long history and connection," she said. "I want my family to see that." But she also wanted to be a Moroccan princess on her wedding day, she said, so the following June we had what must have been the first Bedouin-themed wedding with a carpet for an invitation and an orange-and-purple wedding cake in the 250-year history of Mickve Israel synagogue. When Linda told the caterer her fantasy menu, his reaction was, "What's a falafel?"

The next year we set about trying to find time in our busy lives to have children. "You can't time the market," I said, echoing my grandmother's stock market advice, "but you can try!" So we tried, and within weeks we were fortunate to have early positive signs. Linda went to the store to buy a home pregnancy test. The instructions said to pee on the paper, and if one pink strip appears, you are not pregnant; if two pink strips appear, you are.

The first time, Linda got one pink strip and one faint, *half-pink* strip. We didn't know what that meant. She tried again, then the following day, then once more. Every time the same thing. We did a Google search for "pregnancy test" and "half-pink strip." Five hundred and fifty-seven thousand entries appeared. It would seem we had a common problem.

Finally Linda went to three separate drugstores and came back with an armful of pregnancy tests. I joked that being married to a woman who went to Harvard and Yale meant I had a wife who had to pass *every pregnancy test ever made*. She wasn't satisfied until she found one that said, simply: PREGNANT. Then, we knew.

Then she started throwing up. Not once a day, but twice a day. Sometimes three. Unlike me, who gets food poisoning at the drop of a kebab, Linda hadn't vomited since childhood, so the experience unnerved her. I sat on the tub and tried to comfort her. We bought saltines by the case. Over time, she began to accept, even laugh at, the relentlessness. For a high-flying executive, it was an adjustment for her to be patient and let her baby be in control. This was her first lesson in motherhood.

At about eight and a half weeks, we went to see an OB. A young woman walked in, gave us a thick folder, and patiently answered our questions. Then it was time for the sonogram. Linda mounted the spread-eagled chair, and soon an indecipherable gray image appeared on the screen. The doctor was silent for the longest time before she said with a slight hiccup in her voice, "Well, my dear, you're having, um, twins." Then she added, "Disregard everything I've told you up to now."

It would be safe to say that Linda and I are both talkers. But we were silent at this news. We had never contemplated having twins. Never discussed it. Never even considered discussing it. The popular notion is that twins run in the family; neither of us has twins in our immediate families. The other common cause of twins is fertility drugs; we weren't using fertility drugs.

But we were having twins.

Or maybe not. The doctor explained that our twins appeared to be in the same sac, a potentially dangerous condition in which one fetus is likely to deprive the other of nutrition. Within seconds we heard a chilling expression: "selective reduction." Minutes later we were in a taxi on our way to the highest floor of the city's largest hospital to be screened by New York's most powerful sonogram. "The joke's on us," Linda said. "We never do things normally!"

"By the way, which is worse?" I added. "Two of you, or two of *me*?"

We laughed.

And then we knew: We would survive only by laughing.

Within hours the sonogram had provided the good news that the girls were in different sacs, and we had moved on to a more specialized doctor. We also began sharing the news with our families. "Linda is pregnant with monochorionic, di-amniotic, naturally conceived identical twins." No one understood what this meant, and, in truth, neither did we. I went to the bookstore and bought a shelfful of volumes, then stayed up half the night devouring them. Most of the news was alarming: A higher risk of miscarriage, a greater chance for birth defects, a significant probability that one fetus sabotages the other. I threw the library into the trash so Linda wouldn't read it.

We began making adjustments and soon were ticking off weeks. Full term for singletons is considered forty weeks; for twins it's thirty-six. A friend who went into premature labor with twins at twenty-six weeks was hospitalized, with her legs elevated, to keep the babies in as long as possible. Our doctor, Mark Gold, was taking no chances. At twenty-five weeks he issued a stark prescription: bed rest. Linda was confined to our sofa or bed for all but the most extraordinary circumstances. Another way of describing this is house arrest.

Linda's organization by now was operating in seven countries, on three continents, and soon enough she was running it from our couch. Tycoons and philanthropists came to our living room for meetings while I came plodding in in my underwear, bearing food and my cheery reprimand: "Tushy on the cushy!"

At thirty-six weeks I bought Linda a chocolate-and-peanut-butter cake and graffitied her stomach exactly the same way I had forbidden my mother to do to my cast years earlier. We hastened our search for names. My mother always joked that she had named my siblings and me like hurricanes—Andrew, Bruce, and Cari. But we were actually named after relatives, as was customary among American Jews at the time. Bruce Stephen honored my maternal grandfather, Benjamin "Bucky" Samuel Abeshouse, who had died three years before my birth.

I didn't much like my name growing up. I found it too white bread and too assimilationist. So Linda and I went in the opposite direction. We turned to the Hebrew Bible, but the selection of biblical girls' names is thin. I was in Turkey, wading in the Euphrates, while taping a television show about the Garden of Eden, when Linda proposed that one of our girls be named Eden. It sounded familiar and exotic, feminine yet strong.

We spent the next six months trying to find a match for it. As travelers, we particularly liked that Eden was a place, a paradise. One day, Linda blurted out, "What about Tybee?" A barrier island off the coast of Georgia, Tybee is a place where the Feilers have spent summers for four generations. It's also something of an anti-paradise. "Seedy Savannah Beach" we called it growing up. But all of us, especially Linda, have come to treasure it.

Still the name posed problems. Adding one name that is easily mispronounced—Tybee, which rhymes with "my bee"—to another—Feiler, which rhymes with "Tyler"— seemed foolhardy. Also, Tybee is the Creek Indian word meaning "salt." Not exactly the stuff of love songs. Finally, Linda prevailed. "She'll be interesting," she said of our daughter. "She'll be able to handle it."

———

AT THIRTY-EIGHT WEEKS, WE visited Lenox Hill hospital for our latest sonogram. Linda had gained fifty pounds, almost entirely around her midsection. She looked as if she were carrying a planet under her orange shirt. The radiologist explained that there was a great debate about how long to carry twins: let them stay in as long as possible, or bring them out when they're cooked. "I'm in the latter camp," he said. He glanced at the screen, then announced in a voice that made it clear he was looking for any excuse to support his cause, "Oooh, I see something. . . . You don't have enough fluid! You're having your babies tomorrow."

Our hearts raced. We went for a stroll down Park Avenue, where daffodils bobbed like chicks and tulips sprouted like fistfuls of crayons.

At 8:30 A.M. on April 15, Linda was induced. By noon her water had broken. By late afternoon she had gone into labor. Just after 5:00 P.M., we proceeded into the operating room. "Push! Push! Push!" the nurses shouted as they rolled the gurney down the hall. And as they struggled with the bed, we shouted back, "Push, push, push!" We all laughed.

"Keep it down!" The chief nurse scowled from her station. "There's far too much laughter for a hospital."

Linda and I looked at each other. We wanted our daughters to be born into laughter!

Inside the operating room, the atmosphere was more sober. About fifteen people were crowded into the huddle of monitors, fluorescent lights, plastic incubators, and heat lamps. Linda's hair was netted. Dr. Gold disappeared between her legs, and the nurses gathered around her head. Two heartbeats *thump-thumped* a steady soundtrack. For months, one of our girls had been closer to the cervix and thus earned the moniker Twin A, meaning she was expected to come out first. But Twin B was more active, and as Linda predicted, at the last moment she pushed her sister out of the way and, at 6:14 P.M., made her way first into the world. She was the saltier of the two. She was Tybee Rose.

I was called over to hold her. She was wrapped in a white blanket with blue stripes. Her skin was dark; her hair almost black. She reminded me of her mother. I began to whisper a poem into her ear. As I did, chaos erupted on the far side of the room.

For years I'd heard friends say that the moment they first held their son or daughter was one of the highlights of their lives, like looking into the face of God. But in my case, God was distracted. Linda was in pain. Twin A was in trouble.

I suddenly felt torn between the baby in my arms and my wife on the table. The choice was clear. This was the moment I learned that with twins, there is no such thing as unbifurcated emotion. You don't get a moment with one that doesn't have the shadow of the other.

"The heartbeat is sinking," Dr. Gold said. "Time to scrub."

As soon as he spoke, I realized why so many people were in the room. There was an entire surgical team prepared to give Linda a C-section in the event something went wrong. Linda had said for months that she didn't care if her babies were delivered naturally or by caesarean. But she was adamant that she didn't want one of each, thus doubling her side effects and recovery time. She was now facing this scenario.

"No!" barked the head nurse, who was wrapped around Linda's neck. "I think she can do it."

And with that Linda began to push harder. I later learned that threatening the mother of twins with a C-section is an old obstetric trick to get her to push out the second baby, but Dr. Gold insisted he wasn't playing that game. Whatever the case, it worked. Thirty-two minutes after the birth of her sister, Twin B came sliding down after her. Eden Elenor completed our family.

Linda held up two fingers and beamed. She had carried our daughters for thirty-eight weeks and delivered them naturally within the same hour. I leaned over and touched my forehead to hers. "You did it, baby," I whispered. "Twenty fingers and twenty toes."

I went over to hold Eden. The stripes on her blanket were green. Her skin and hair seemed fairer. She looked more like me. I whispered in her ear the same poem I had recited to her sister. By the time I returned to Linda's side, Dr. Gold was stitching her up. Suddenly, he looked down at his watch.

"Hmmm," he said. "Tax day. Early Feiler and Late Feiler."

And with that our daughters were welcomed into their lives with a roomful of laughter.

·4·

CHRONICLES OF THE LOST YEAR

volume I

July 15

Dear Friends and Family,

The mist lifts slowly off my in-laws' back lawn on Cape Cod most mornings, revealing a day that is well under way and a layer of dew on the granite boulders. The sky has been gray over Snug Harbor the last few days, but at last the clouds have magically parted and the air turned sunny once more.

I apologize for reaching out in this way, but the crush of events in recent days has forced us into a number of uncomfortable situations. I have learned that I have a seven-inch osteogenic sarcoma in my left femur.

Put more directly: I have bone cancer. My sarcoma is considered very rare, and very aggressive. It has already eaten through the central shaft of my bone and corroded large portions of the thigh muscle around it. My knee and hip appear to be safe, and early signs that the cancer may have spread to my ribs and lungs have been downplayed. We believe it's contained to my leg, but the situation continues to be very fluid and could change at any time.

The tumor was discovered by accident after a routine blood test in late May produced an elevated alkaline phosphatase number, a nonspecific test indicating possible problems in the liver or bones. My liver was cleared, and a series of tests led us to where we are now. One remarkable aspect of my situation is that I am, for the most part, pain free. This type of tumor usually presents itself through pain, swelling, or fracture. In this regard, we are lucky. As one oncologist said to me recently, "Kudos to your internist for discovering your tumor early."

Through the generous and swift intervention of friends, Linda and I had a consultation with Dr. John Healey, the head of orthopedic surgery at Memorial Sloan-Kettering Hospital in New York. Dr. Healey has been variously described to us as "the man," "the one," or "the guru" in this field. He's a genial man in his early fifties with an easy smile, a bow tie, and the unusual-but-arresting

manner of speaking about three words every minute. If
you hang on his every word—and boy do we!—you hang
for a very long time. He also happens to be a fellow
graduate of Ezra Stiles College at Yale University and,
like me, a teenage juggler and clown.

Dr. Healey spent several hours with us and about halfway
through our conversation said of the cancer in my leg:
"In the worst-case scenario, this appears to be curable."
He also said several times, "This is a war, and I intend to
win it."

Dr. Healey thinks my cancer is probably related to the
bicycle accident I had when I was five years old in which
I broke the same bone in the same place. Osteosarcomas
in the femur usually appear closer to the knee or hip;
mine is in the central shaft. We had assumed that the
broken bone did not heal properly, or left behind some
inflammation that somehow cancerified four decades
later. But Dr. Healey hypothesized that the arrow may
point in the opposite direction. When he asked me,
for example, how I had broken my femur, I gave what I
assumed to be the only logical answer: "I was hit by a car."

"But why *that* bone?" he said. He was suggesting that I had
been born with a genetic predisposition that weakened
my left femur.

Regardless, something happened between then and now that made my left femur different from the tens of thousands of other bones children break every year in the United States. And at some point a cell went rogue. A cancer was born. About six hundred Americans get an osteosarcoma every year, and about 85 percent are under the age of twenty-five. Fewer than one hundred adults a year get this disease. (Compare that with 200,000 cases of breast cancer a year, or 190,000 cases of prostate cancer.) As a result, very little is known about how to treat this illness, especially in adults. No one wins a Nobel Prize for curing an orphan disease.

Had I faced this diagnosis twenty-five years ago, the doctors would have cut off my leg and hoped. Ted Kennedy's son Teddy lost his leg to this disease when he was twelve. Only 15 percent of patients survived. In the 1980s, doctors discovered that a particular cocktail of chemotherapy was effective, quadrupling the survival rate.

Before proceeding down that route, I must receive a proper analysis of my tumor. I am scheduled to have an open biopsy in the coming weeks, during which Dr. Healey will cut into my leg and extract a piece of the bone. That will be sent for pathology, and then we will begin designing a course of treatment. We have been led to believe that I am likely looking at two to four months of chemotherapy, followed by surgery, followed by four more months of chemotherapy. The surgery will likely involve going into my leg, cutting out the tumor and some additional bone around it, as well as a chunk of muscle. A replacement femur of either cadaver bone or metal will be inserted. The bone will heal, I am told, the muscle will not. If we are fortunate, my leg will be spared, and my knee and foot will function as normal, though my movement will be permanently affected. As Dr. Healey put it, "You will walk, not run. Flat surfaces will be better than stairs."

As you might imagine, this news has hit us with titanic force. After Dr. Healey finished explaining my situation, a nurse came in to have me fill out some forms. I asked her to give Linda and me a few minutes to ourselves. When she left, I broke down on the examination table. I had hoped against hope that I wouldn't have cancer. I had yearned beyond yearning that I could avoid chemotherapy. My hopes were dashed. My yearnings crushed.

I stand at the dawn of a lost year.

At best.

So how are you doing? We're hanging in there. We're focused. We have good spells and bad. We have had plenty of tears and late-night conversations about each other, our lives, and our dreams for our girls. It is not easy. We are not heroes. No one aspires to be the person who handles this kind of situation well. And we don't always handle it well.

Having said that, we have deep resources to draw on—two loving families, many friends, each other, and active minds that lead us both to develop fourteen-point plans for nutritional supplements and to imagine many scenarios, both dire and full of hope. And we have already found occasion to laugh. For instance, why exactly does the examination room of the leading orthopedic cancer surgeon at Sloan-Kettering hospital have a copy of *Tennis Week* at the top of a stack of magazines for patients to read?

How is Linda? A star. One of the first casualties of this news was a trip to Nantucket we had planned to celebrate our fifth anniversary. It was to be our first without the girls since they were born three years ago. Linda swallowed, teared up, took a breath, and moved on. As anyone who has been through one of these situations knows, the burden is invariably hardest on the spouse, caregiver, or "co-survivor" as they are sometimes called. Linda will have many challenges balancing her work, the needs of the girls, and an intermittently grumpy, perpetually gimpy husband (OK, so the grumpy has been there all along, but the gimpy is new!). Chemo is fun for no one.

With that said, Linda's nonprofit, Endeavor, is
thriving. Last year the organization marked ten years/
ten countries of helping entrepreneurs around the
world, and Endeavor is poised to receive a generous
grant from a private foundation in the coming weeks
that will accelerate its growth. I can say with conviction
that it is extremely important to me personally that
Linda continue to devote as much time as possible to
her inspiring work and continue to make some of the
handful of international trips she has planned in the
coming months. Life will change, but it cannot stop. In
that spirit, I would like to ask anyone reading these words
to join me in ways large and small to help keep Linda's
spirits up and to help her continue to give off the light
she does to so many.

How are the girls? Eden and Tybee are also thriving.
Turning three proved to be the moment when the gender
switch flipped, and they are deeply focused on ballet,
as well as princesses, cupcakes, and all things pink and
purple. Actually, they are focused on one particular
pink leotard and one chosen pair of purple "footed
tights." Three years of parental determination to bypass
traditional gender color coding was summarily tossed
down the pastel fairy hole. In the last few weeks the girls
went bowling, boating, and played miniature golf—all for
the first time. And at least one of those activities may be
for the last: When Papa Alan, who's just getting the hang

of his new motorboat, decided to merely put-put around
the harbor and shy away from the open seas, Eden
quickly blurted out, "When are we going to go *faster*?!"

We have been consulting with experts on how and what
to tell the girls about my illness, and early indications
are to be honest but nonspecific and have everyone repeat
the same line: "Daddy is sick. The doctors are helping
him. He's going to get better." Then we will watch like
hawks to see if there is any change in behavior, including
a lack of focus, increased aggression, or nightmares.
They already see that Daddy is on crutches, and we can
watch them adjusting. When Linda and I rejoined them
on Cape Cod this week after a few days consulting with
doctors in New York, Eden said, "I'm so happy you
comed back." We are proud of them, we love them, and
I look forward to walking them down the aisle someday
and to leading them on short walks, at least, around the
world.

What can I do to help? We are very grateful for the many
people who have asked this question, and the honest
answer is that we're trying to think through how
to provide guidance that is truthful, realistic, and
meaningful—and respects the genuine emotion behind
it. We're already finding that giving people specific
things can be helpful—"Hey, Ma, I need a shower
stool"; "Hey, Sis, we need a three-ring binder for all the

paperwork"; "Hey, Bro, can you take some pictures of me before I lose my hair." If you give us some time to suss out more completely what we're facing, we'd love to have your support.

That's the view from week one. I have been overwhelmed by the many e-mails and calls that have already started to come in. We read every one. Please know that the onslaught of doctor consultations, insurance negotiations, crappy days, and glimmers of clarity in which I try to find some productivity or study the origins of a grand plié might mean I don't have time to write you back, but your thoughtfulness will continue to give me comfort and strength. It is my intention to send out regular letters in the coming months to update you on my progress.

In the meantime, may you find clear skies out your window this summer, may your arrows all point forward, and may you find your way onto the open water sometime soon going just as fast as you want.

Until then, take a walk for me.

Love,

Bruce

5

JEFF

Approach the Cow

THE DUNGEON DISCO IN THE Castle Assumburg youth hostel in northern Holland was blaring Michael Jackson and throbbing with red lights as I slipped out the back door and stared at the cow farm just over the moat. It was the summer of 1983, a few weeks after my high school graduation, and I was just beginning a six-week student exchange program in Europe. My first trip abroad, the tour was a gift from my grandmother and would lead us through the Netherlands, Germany, Italy, Switzerland, and France. It was Tuesday, so to speak, so we were in Holland.

Not exactly a disco goer, I had snuck out the serfs' entrance and was soon joined by our coleader, Jeff, whose parents had started this student travel company thirty-two years earlier in Putney, Vermont. Tall, lanky, with an angular nose and a boyish bowl of brown hair, Jeff could alternate between the hick Vermont farmer who loved to shovel manure and the cosmopolitan French-speaking college senior whose mother was Dutch and whose father grew up amid the footlights of Broadway. Mostly he was an imp, with a wicked sense of adventure, and he could tell I was just naive and untraveled enough to be a perfect foil for his evangelical mischievousness.

"Ever been cow tipping?" he asked.

"Cow what?" I said.

"Cows sleep standing up, so if you sneak up on them upwind, you can push them over and they'll make a giant thud on the ground."

Before I could figure out if he was making this up, we had jumped the moat, scaled the barbed wire, squished through the mud and patties of dung, and were just about to approach some poor dozing cow.

And I had discovered the great passion of my life: the unexpected, never-ending university of travel.

———

I almost didn't tell Linda about my idea of a Council of Dads. It would be too upsetting for her to imagine; too morbid to consider. We should focus on the positive. We should live in the moment. But within twenty-four hours I had lost my resolve, and as soon as I described my still unformed conception, the idea no longer belonged just to me. It was ours, somehow. Really, it was hers, because Linda was the one who might someday be called on to choreograph the relationships between these dads and our girls.

Yet even after I conceded that her views carried more weight than mine, we soon twisted ourselves into knots. "I love him," she would say of a prospective dad, "but he doesn't represent who you are now." "He's great," she would add of another, "but what about *this* part of you."

We needed a set of guidelines.

First, no family members. The man I'm closest to in the world is my brother. I also have brothers-in-law, cousins, and the like with whom I share any number of bonds. But we figured these men would naturally have relationships with our girls and would share in family occasions throughout their lives.

Second, men only. I have been blessed since I was a teenager with unusually strong friendships with women; my list of closest friends would probably be split fifty-fifty. But we concluded that with their mother still in their lives, what our girls would need were fatherly voices to fill the vacuum of my absence.

Third, intimacy over longevity. We decided that some of my more recent friendships might better capture the man I had become and father I wanted to be.

Fourth, only one friend from each phase of my life.

And finally, a dad for every side. We didn't set out

with a preconceived number—and didn't care whether the men were fathers themselves—but instead looked for men who might capture different aspects of my personality. As Linda kept repeating, "I want men I can call when I face some challenge and the girls come to me and ask, 'What would Daddy think of this?'" In the end we chose men who embodied parts of me.

———

AND FROM THE BEGINNING, Jeff Shumlin was on the list.

In the decades since we first stepped into that cow patch, Jeff and I had strengthened our bond. He and his brother eventually took over their parents' student travel business. Jeff settled in bucolic Putney, married a photographer, and had two children. He volunteered as a fireman, served as a selectman, spent part of every day riding around on his tractor, and, yup, shoveled manure.

And for me, Putney became a sort of storybook playground, a place where I went to chop wood, pick apples, and tap maple syrup. It was a place where Jeff's neighbor stood in the barn, sliced a breath mint with his pocketknife, and stuck a piece in the gap of his front teeth. It was a place where the general store sold Chef Boyardee and Yoo-hoos and made me feel like Homer Price and his doughnut machine. It was a place I went after every breakup and bad review.

And Jeff became that friend from the summer I grew up. He was my camp counselor: racing me to the top of mountains, throwing me in the lake, nearly shooting me in the head when a deer jumped from behind a tree and leapt over my Elmer Fudd hat. He was my life coach: pushing me to study abroad, hectoring me to marry Linda. He was my big brother, the one whom I always looked up to, because I wanted to, because he deserved it.

And when I got sick, Jeff was the one who started sending me a postcard, every day, snow or shine, vacation or work, and vowed to continue for as long as I was ill.

It was this mixture of qualities I wanted Jeff to convey to our girls: the connectedness of someone who understood the value of neighbors, along with the openness of someone who spent half his life living and working in other parts of the world. Jeff would show the girls how to engage their community, then carry that way to experience life with them around the globe.

Jeff would teach them how to travel.

So a few weeks after my diagnosis, we loaded the car, packed up the girls, and made the drive up Route 91 to our farm away from home in Vermont. That afternoon, Jeff took our girls for a ride on the John Deere, then led them on a chase after runaway pigs. Afterward, he and I drove to an abandoned barn overlooking an apple orchard, with a stretch of green hills in the distance. We set up a pair of beach chairs. "The best thing I can do is read this," I said. I took a deep breath and began to read my letter to the dads. Tears mottled my voice, and I could barely complete the words.

Will you help be their dad?

Will you be my voice.

I suddenly felt old. Yet I also felt secure. Mostly, as I watched his eyes well up and his body stiffen, I felt sad to be burdening him with my pain.

Then the letter was over and the view before us no longer seemed beautiful. The ground had become almost a burial spot. We were two travelers arrived in a place where we didn't want to belong.

"Yes," Jeff said, answering the request that I had forgotten was in my letter. "I'd be honored." He paused. "But I'm not a man of words. I'm a dad by example."

Suddenly my idea was no longer just mine. And no longer Linda's, either.

It was his, too.

It had life.

GEORGE SHUMLIN WAS A high school English teacher in Putney in 1949 when he sailed home from a summer in Europe. One night a huge storm rocked the *Nieuw Amsterdam,* and most of the passengers fled to sleep. "Even the bartenders were sick," Jeff explained. "My father went looking for people to play cards. One of them was my mother, who was studying in British Columbia. She also had a strong stomach and knew how to play bridge." The next summer the two spent a week together in Paris; the following year the head of George's school proposed they lead a group of students to Europe. The only catch: They had to get married or they would set a poor example. They had spent fewer than ten days together.

"They went off to do something fun that summer and quickly realized the value of experiential learning," Jeff said. "And that very much became the core of our philosophy. Growth through a sense of community; immersion as the key to learning." Within a few years Kitty and George started Putney Student Travel, which in time grew to include hundreds of students. As soon as Jeff and his siblings were born, they were thrust into the family business. "My father would drive to New York and see off every group," Jeff said. "He would make a speech at the Barbizon Plaza Hotel on Central Park South while we ran crazy in the back of the room."

"So what did he say?"

"He talked about the difference between mass travel, where everybody is isolated in buses, and really getting off the beaten track: taking risks, living with families, doing things that are uncomfortable. My father has a certain gravitas—the way he looks; the way he speaks—and he would set a tone that this was a serious cultural experience."

When Jeff was in college, he was pressed to start leading trips. With his gift for languages and boyish instincts, he was a natural. "Sure, we would touch on big tourist attractions," he said, "but I also knew how to turn left down some little alley and lead the kids to some undiscovered part of Paris, or put them on bicycles and hop out to the beach in Brittany and make a bonfire at night with a bunch of French kids."

"What's the value in those?"

"Ask anyone who has traveled and inevitably the most valuable experiences are when pitfalls come up. The day it's rainy and miserable and you get up early to be the first one in line at some museum and you get there and it's closed. You think quickly, you look around, and you go into a tiny hole-in-the-wall café where old men are playing checkers. You get a hot chocolate, you sit down next to them, and you talk about your life. They share theirs. And you have this bonding that you never anticipated, and that is much more valuable than going to the museum and reading the guidebook and listening to the tapes."

Jeff was preparing to lead his third Putney trip in 1983 when I sent in my application.

"You were the perfect foil for my experiential philosophy," Jeff recalled. "First, you were a blank slate. Second, your essay opened with the line 'I am a people person.' From the beginning, when I threw out a crazy idea, you were ready to give it a try. If I tried to lift the spirits of the group by breaking into song—and I'm naturally an inhibited person—you were a great contrast to me because for you the whole world is a stage. You threw open your arms, and before long you and I were singing gospel and other students were diving right in. And we did this while accomplishing some inane task, like climbing off trail up a mountain in the Swiss Alps just because why take the zigzagging trail."

I have two primary memories from that summer, I told him. The first is a string of minor hooliganisms that seemed magical to my buttoned-down, apple-polishing self: cow tipping in Holland; lifting a tiny car in Florence from its parking space and turning it around to face in the opposite direction; sneaking through an open door in the Paris Opera House and sprinting through the underground tunnels in mythical pursuit of the Phantom of the Opera. I asked Jeff what those experiences say.

"It says that the style of leadership I embodied involves a good dose of immaturity!" We laughed. "Seriously, my philosophy has always been: Take the risk. Do something silly. We had no right to be in the back of the Paris Opera House. But if we'd met someone, what an explanation it would have been to say we were just trying to understand the world a little bit. And what if we got thrown out?! It would have been a great story we could all tell our grandchildren. So, seize the opportunity. Turn the car around. Approach the cow."

My second memory involves a week I spent with a family in Groningen, Holland. My first night, after a startlingly white meal of fish, potatoes, and yogurt, the family retired to the television, and I retreated to the water closet. There was only one problem: I couldn't figure out how to flush the toilet. There was no handle, no button, no lever, no rope. The tank was located near the ceiling, and I decided to flush the toilet manually. I stood on the lid, reached up toward the tank, and was just about to remove the cover, when . . . there was a knock on the door.

"Are you okay?" someone inquired.

"Um, I'm fine!" I sang.

The family shuffled back to the living room, but their teenage daughter leaned close to the door and whispered, "Pull down the pipe!" That night I cried myself to sleep. A week later, after biking the nearby dunes and stuffing liverwurst into muslin casings in a butcher's basement, I had forged such a deep connection with the family that when it was time to leave, the daughter and her friends came to the train station with a giant American flag and sang "The Star-Spangled Banner" as we pulled out.

"That story would bring tears to my father's eyes," Jeff said, "because it's the crux of his speech on Central Park South. 'It's not going to be easy. It's going to take adjustment. But get your hands dirty, go into the basement, and stuff liver into a sack. Be a traveler, not a tourist.'"

"So what is a traveler?" I asked.

"A traveler is someone who can let go of what is familiar and in a very conscious way seek out what is different. It is someone willing to slow down enough, get off the pressured, achievement track, and seize the opportunity. It is someone willing to break the routines of home: what you eat, when you sleep, how you wash."

He went on. "It's meeting the cheese maker in a village, and before long you're in the barn up to your elbows in whey. It's sleeping on a dirt floor in Tanzania, using a pit latrine, screaming every time you see a bug, then realizing that the people who live there, the ones who carry water in a bucket for miles, are just as happy, if not more so, than you are. It's being at a reception in Afghanistan, eating unidentifiable food, then discovering later that it was goat's stomach, and that the animal was slaughtered in your honor by people who simply appreciated the ability to interact with you."

The afternoon had slipped into evening by now. Our families were waiting back at the house. We sat up in our chairs.

"So it's ten years from now," I said. "We've gathered at the Barbizon Plaza Hotel, and our daughters are about to leave on their first trip abroad. You've earned the gravitas that your father always had, and—I'll say it—I'm not there." For a second, the emotion of why we had gathered returned to my voice. "What will you say to my girls?"

He took a deep breath. "I think I would say, 'Girls, you come from a background that's open to the world. You come from a set of values that appreciates learning, and you will have many opportunities to take in human civilization at its highest levels of achievement. But I would urge you to approach this experience as a small child might approach a mud puddle. You can lean over and look at yourself in the reflection, maybe stick a finger in it, and cause a little ripple. Or you can dive in, thrash around, and find out what it feels like, what it tastes like. . . .' "

Once again Jeff had the same twinkle in his eye I first saw that night behind the castle in Holland. He had that look that said, "Hey, let's go cow tipping," even though we never did actually tip the cow. Even though no one tips the cow. Even though cows don't sleep standing up.

" 'I urge you to jump in, girls,' " he said. " 'And I look forward to seeing you, back here, at the end of this experience, covered in mud.' "

6

TWENTIETH-CENTURY
TWO-THIRDS

M Y BROTHER KNEW THE GUN was there. My father sensed that his father was feeling down. My mother believed he needed an outlet other than work.

Just before lunchtime, on Wednesday, March 30, 1983, Edwin J. Feiler stood at his dresser on Early Street, immediately behind our home on Lee Boulevard, and scribbled a note to his family. Then he strolled into the bathroom with the gold and white tile. For as long as anyone could remember, my grandfather and grand-mother had slept in separate bedrooms. It was a South-ern thing, perhaps, a nod to gentility from the traveling salesman's son who rose to become a small-town law-yer. It was a mark of formality for a man who earned an honorary title from the governor and told my stupefied, Baltimore-born mother, "Just call me 'Colonel.'"

Or maybe it was the manifestation of a pain he could never express.

"I spent two hours with him that morning," recalled Jazie Ingram, his bookkeeper. "His Parkinson's was getting worse; he was showing signs of dementia. 'I'll never come back to the office,' he told me. I said, 'Sure, you will!' But now I realize he was sending me a message."

Standing in the bathroom, he surely couldn't avoid looking in the mirror. He would have seen a once-jolly face with spectacles, a teardrop nose, and a gap between his two front teeth. Perhaps he paused. Twelve days later he would turn seventy-eight. A month later I would graduate from high school. The following year he would celebrate fifty years of marriage.

He put the pistol to his temple.

My grandmother was a few steps away in the den. She heard the gunshot. She found her husband folded on the floor. He was still alive. She reached my dad on the telephone. "Your father shot himself. There's a lot of blood." My dad hurried to the hospital. "He'll never recover," the doctor told him. My father made the decision to grant his father's wish. It was he who ended his dad's life.

"He thought he was doing it to relieve the burden on all of us," my father said. "Instead he gave us a burden for the rest of our lives."

THE TAPE WAS SCRATCHY after all these years, but the voice was slow, clear, and strong. It reminded me of white corn in summer, a bit of old country charm.

> *This is to be the story of the life of Edwin Jacob Feiler, born in Meridian, Mississippi, on April 11, 1905. I am going to call it* Twentieth-Century Two-thirds. *The reason for this is that I have lived and been active for approximately the first two-thirds of the twentieth century. That is from 1905 until the present date, 1970.*

From 1970 to 1982, my grandfather recorded twenty-eight cassette tapes that detailed his childhood, his education, and his sometimes-colorful professional rise. He was a notoriously slow driver in the brown Ford Granada he owned during most of those years, and he dictated as he drove. After the suicide, my father had the tapes transcribed. The resulting document, four-hundred-plus pages, sat in the family vault, unread, for more than two decades.

That is, until I got sick.

Faced with my own mortality, I suddenly ached to know why Papa had ended his life. I was curious if the tapes might answer some long-held questions I harbored about his life. Mostly I wondered if his memoirs contained clues about our family that might benefit my girls. In a year in which I was trying to capture my own

voice for my daughters, I first had to revisit the voices
that had fed into mine.

———

EDWIN JACOB FEILER WAS raised in a modest frame
house in Meridian, Mississippi, a railroad town near the
Alabama border. The house had no central heat and no
hot water heater. "By the time I came along they had
electric lights," he noted. The highlight of the week was
when ice arrived by freight train because it meant he
could order a cold Coca-Cola at the drugstore.

The Feilers were descended from a wave of German Jews who had emigrated to the United States in the
mid-nineteenth century, bypassed New York, and headed
deep into the South. Many of these families went into
the grocery and dry goods business, and Papa's father,
Melvin, was a traveling salesman for one such firm. He
never made more than $250 a month, his son recalled,
and "never had any money that he considered a gain or
a surplus."

The principal lesson my grandfather took from his
father's plight was the same one he passed on to us as
we drove with him on Saturday morning to work in the
family office. The proper life is the working life. The
highest value is labor. The one treasure no one can ever
take away from you is the self-confidence from knowing
you have done a good and earnest job.

And boy did he do a good job—in dozens of unglamorous circumstances. From the time he could throw a baseball, my grandfather was working. He collected payments for a dry cleaner, he sold penny magazines, he delivered scenery to the opera house (and hung around to ogle the actresses). He delivered homemade medicines from Stanley's Drug Company, namely, stomach tonic, which was 98 percent alcohol, and hair tonic, which was 99. "I didn't realize at the time that Prohibition was what brought about the sale of all these tonics."

He was consumed with self-improvement. He went to the library and read the entire *World Book Encyclopedia*. He reveled in every good grade and teacher's praise. On the one-year anniversary of the armistice of World War I, a group of students decided to take an unannounced day off. "That was their fatal mistake," my grandfather recalls. "I had no more idea of walking away from that school than flying." The renegade students were suspended for two weeks, and "practically everyone failed their courses."

My grandfather attended the University of Georgia, then law school, where he earned a spot in Phi Kappa Phi for being in the top 10 percent. He briefly joined the army, then moved to Savannah. Renting a room in the YMCA, he was disheartened to find little demand—or respect—for lawyers. So he did what he did best: He adapted. He wrote wills; he sprung people from jail; he defended gangsters and pornographers. And he got breaks. A steamship went down in the Atlantic, and he handled the claims. He got a coveted job defending the railroads against a law that held them responsible for any cow found dead within twenty feet of a railroad. Someone, it seems, *was* cow tipping, and it was the Southern and Coastline railways.

By the time my father joined him in 1959, and they pioneered the business of low-income loans, little Eddie Feiler had finally achieved some of the status he long craved. "I have dwelt on the things that were successful," he says near the end of the tapes, "and purposefully left off the things that weren't. Nobody wants to be bored with my troubles. They get bored enough with my successes!"

———

BUT AS I READ, I sensed a darker, sometimes sadder story infused with his successes.

For starters, he was remarkably candid about the seamy side of small-town life. He describes bags of cash being passed around the police department and the judges' chambers. He includes a recipe for brewing moonshine. And when the army plans a base near Savannah, he and a friend drive all day to Columbus, to investigate how soldiers spend their pay. My grandfather brings along my dad, then five, but leaves him in the hotel—alone!— when they go out to inspect the layout of local brothels. "When I got home and told my wife," he reports, "I was the recipient of considerable scorn."

Even more haunting, an air of premature, spectacular death shadows his life. His earliest memory is the sinking of *Titanic*. The first time he sees a plane, at the Mississippi State Fair, it crashes and kills the pilot. Later, when a firm in Pittsburgh suggests he and a colleague fly up for a meeting, my grandfather declines, declaring the plane unsafe. His friend chose to fly, and the airplane crashed, claiming his life.

More troubling, my grandfather could recount exacting details of bank failures and equity trades. His memoirs are so dry in places that when he mentions coming to Tybee Island to visit our family, I felt a well of relief. But in twenty-eight tapes, in *twelve years of recording his life,* he never describes his mother—or what he felt about her. He doesn't talk about his sister. He never mentions his wife by name—or their courtship or wedding. My father is referred to fewer than half a dozen times; his younger brother even less. My mother does not appear at all, my brother and I only once, my sister never. Women come up only when he describes how difficult it was to hire good secretaries.

A son of the dirt-poor South, my grandfather surely loved his family. But his complete disinterest in personal feelings was undeniable—and maybe the clue I had been seeking all these years. He simply didn't define himself by relationships. He was that boy looking for work; that young, hungry lawyer; the man on the rise. I had always believed that he could have relieved his pain if he had someone to talk to in those final years. But his memoir told me he had a deeper problem: He had no one to listen to him at all. He felt alone in the world.

And maybe that's why, when he did come down with Parkinson's, when he could no longer be productive, when he lost his sense of self, he ignored the feelings of his wife sitting in the next room, of his son building their business, of his grandson about to reach a milestone.

His work had come to an end.

He had no other reason to live.

———

AFTER THE AMBULANCE LEFT for the hospital, Jazie Ingram went to 333 Early Street to clean up the blood my grandfather had discharged all over the bathroom tile.

"I loved him," she explained. "He was like a second father to me." She and I were sitting in his former office, which Jazie has used for the last quarter century. No taller than an ice-cream sundae, Jazie speaks with the cane-syrup sweetness (and occasional rattlesnake bite) of her rural Baptist upbringing. "I have something you might want to see," she said.

She walked into the vault and returned moments later with a piece of paper. It was yellowed with time and stained with pain. The words were large, as if written by a child.

I cannot live a sick man. I am taking my own
life. Edwin J. Feiler

His life ended where it had always been lived: With
one last piece of work. His final act was conscientious,
professional, and cool. It was devoid of emotion.

"There's one thing I want you to hear," Jazie said.
"Even though it was a month before you graduated from
high school, I know your grandfather was proud of you.
He loved you. You must know that."

I sat there frozen, unable to speak. Tears poured
down my cheeks. I hadn't gone seeking confirmation,
but now I realized I must have been waiting for it all
along.

And sitting in my grandfather's office, I began to
see how my own experience with sickness had changed
how I viewed my grandfather's death, and with it the
role of being male in my family. Like many men of his
time—particularly men of the South—Papa approached
his illness as a saddle to bear, both wordlessly and alone.
He didn't even share his anxieties with his family. I, by
contrast, was not only writing regular letters to family
and friends, but I was also sending them through e-mail,
which meant they were being bounced around to people
I didn't even know.

Papa never talked about his feelings. I talked of
nothing else.

And as someone trying to figure out how to "live a

sick man," I suddenly yearned to be transported back to that bedroom where he slept without his wife, to that dresser where he scribbled that note, to that mirror where he stared at himself for the final time, to be able to call out across the generations what the men who came after him have been able to learn.

"We're listening, Papa. We hear you.

"You are not alone."

7

CHRONICLES OF THE LOST YEAR

volume II

August 15

Dear Friends and Family,

Some rain passed through Brooklyn in the last week, leaving us with a string of clear, beautiful afternoons. The Brooklyn Bridge, which just turned 125 years old, is looking fresh-faced and handsome overhead, its famed promenade glittering like the pot of gold at the end of a long journey to come.

On July 31, I was admitted to Memorial Sloan-Kettering Hospital in Manhattan for the first of a dozen cycles of chemotherapy. Each cycle lasts one to three weeks. Because initial exposure to chemotherapy can trigger heart failure, I was kept at the hospital as a precaution. After what seemed like a month of anticipation, followed by a banquet of pills, a nurse hooked my arm up to an IV of Cisplatin and unwrapped three syringes of Adriamycin. The liquid in the syringes was the consistency of melted lollipops and the color of a Shirley Temple. I whispered to the drugs, "Be good to me," then closed my eyes. Tears pushed against the inside of my eyelids. I didn't want Linda to see me cry. What these drugs do to my body over the next three-quarters of a year will go a long way toward shaping the rest of my life: How long it lasts; how much quality I take out of it; whether I have one at all. The nurse noticed I was having a reaction.

"Are you okay?" she asked.

"Physically, yes. Emotionally, it's just very intense."

"Don't worry," she said. "These drugs are going to make you better."

The biopsy on my left femur had confirmed that I have a high-grade, osteoblastic, osteogenic sarcoma. As my surgeon, Dr. Healey, put it, "You have a bad disease." Pediatric sarcomas appearing in adults are extremely rare, with a 30 to 40 percent chance of recurrence in the lungs in the first five years. The morning I heard those figures was one of the worst of my life.

At the same time, these tumors are responsive to chemotherapy and in many cases can be cured outright. My doctors agree that the seven-inch tumor in my left femur will not kill me; it's eventually coming out; but the cancer cells that have likely spread to my blood and are looking for trouble are the graver threat. For that reason, we are leaving the tumor in place for now.

My oncologist is Dr. Robert Maki of Sloan-Kettering. Bean-pole tall with aw-shucks reserve, he has the unfortunate quality of reminding some people of me (at least in appearance, and some pounds ago at that). If Dr. Healey is the rousing warrior, straight out of *The Iliad*, Dr. Maki is the upstanding do-gooder—think Gregory Peck as a young Abe Lincoln. He has called for four to six months of aggressive chemo, followed by surgery in which the bulk of my femur will be removed and replaced, followed by three more months of chemo, then extensive physical therapy. The Lost Year.

A lot of the specifics of treatment will be determined by how a forty-three-year-old man bounces back from a course of treatment used much more often in teenagers. As many of you have sadly learned, the idea behind chemotherapy is to flood the bloodstream with poison, which the more aggressive, rapidly dividing cells in your body hungrily attack. This includes not only malignant cancers, but also hair and the lining of the gastrointestinal tract. My particular chemo drugs are also neurotoxic, meaning they assault the central nervous system. The body's reaction is to rally around the vital organs to protect them, thus leaving more peripheral parts to suffer. I am therefore vulnerable to permanent hearing loss, as well as numbness in my fingers and toes. The resulting list of dos and don'ts is quite precise, including no sushi, manicures, or tattoos. Really, how do metrosexual Japanese bikers get through this?!

On the side-effect front, my first week after taking the drugs was pretty brutal, with an ever-changing menu of nausea, heartburn, dry mouth, fatigue, and a smog in my head as thick as that over Mexico City. I probably sat up in bed less than one hour a day; ate only half a bowl of chicken soup and a cup of Jell-O; and grunted through the few phone conversations I was forced to have. With the fog in my brain, I would have had a difficult time picking out my daughters in a ballet lineup. I feared I would not leave my bed until Valentine's Day.

After bottoming out around Day 7, my energy and appetite returned astonishingly strong. In my second week, I've coordinated over a dozen relatives moving up and down the East Coast to help us out; supervised home renovations; and eaten a Michael Phelps–size diet of barbecue, tacos, and Graeter's cherry ice cream from Cincinnati. I have a third week to regain my strength before being walloped again.

So how have you all been reacting? Depends on when you get us, frankly. Our families have lurched into action, and my parents, in-laws, siblings, and cousins have helped us manage the house and the girlies. Much of the brunt of all this falls on Linda, who not only has a husband retching in the bathroom many nights at 2:00 A.M. but two darling daughters who have yet to fully grasp the meaning of: "Please play in your room until the digital clock says 7:00 A.M.!" Then, just when I hit the nadir, Linda came down with a case of shingles, forcing her to be quarantined in a nearby hotel for three days. As she said of this stress-related illness, "Message: I care!"

The girls have been adapting to our new lifestyle. In a bid to show them that losing my hair was an affirmative choice, as opposed to a negative reaction from the medicine, I had my head shaved like a marine. They were instantly charmed by my "shoft" hair, their homemade combination of *short* and *soft*. In one of the more amusing sideshows around here, their grandmothers had the idea of feeding them a diet of films with bald, father-hero types to prepare them for the inevitable hair loss to come. To date, this has included Daddy Warbucks from *Annie* and was about to include King Mongkut from *The King and I* until someone pointed out that he dies at the end of the movie.

In the early weeks, Eden and Tybee did show signs of

empathy and stress. They stared intently at my new crutches, trying to figure out how they worked and what they meant. Eden suddenly had the need for multiple Band-Aids; Tybee started to limp every now and then. We had some bed-wetting and the occasional nightmare.

A few nights ago, at 4:30 A.M., Eden went over to Tybee's bed and started jumping up and down on the mattress. Linda got up to deal with this unusual outbreak but was quickly flustered. By the time I hobbled down the hall, Eden was on the potty, Tybee was crying, and general chaos had ensued. I tried every trick I know: Threatening. Offering "grown-up" points. Volunteering to tell a story. No dent. Worse: Tybee wanted to listen to Brazilian sambas and Eden wanted Disney love songs.

At this point, I lost it: I snapped at Linda; I screamed at Tybee; I picked up Eden and plunked her down on her bed. Then I began to sob. This was my worst nightmare writ large. My illness was ruining the lives of everyone around me. Linda was suffering. The girls were unraveling. I was a wreck. Our home had become a gruesome parade of psychological disfigurement.

I left the room. "If you want to speak to me," I blurted to Eden, "come to my office." To my utter shock, five minutes later she followed. I sat on the floor, and she climbed into my lap, perching on my right leg. I tried to perform some archaeology on her feelings. First she was mad at her sister. Then her mommy. Then she unfolded this story: Monsters have invaded our house, she said. They sit with us at dinner and eat us up. "Then we are lost," she said, "because we can't walk."

Walk. The word leapt out of the story like a mushroom cloud. Walking had been such a hallmark around our house. Walking is what Daddy did. Even before they could walk themselves, Linda taught the girls that I had written a book about walking. Now, walking is exactly what I could no longer do, and in her nightmare, she couldn't either. I didn't need a Ph.D. in child psychology to understand that she had internalized my illness and created an imaginary situation where the worst that could happen to her was that she would become like me. And what better description of our situation can there be: Monsters *have* invaded our house and are mashing us up.

By now the sun was coming up outside my office window, and Eden's face seemed more tender than I had ever seen it. Her delicate skin sloped gently around her cheeks. The perky lips she inherited from her mother were puckered in fear and need. Her hair bobbed around her face.

I pushed the hair from her eyes, kissed her cheek, and held her close.

"I am going to make the monsters go away," I said. "I have magic and can make our home safe."

She looked down at my leg. "Is this your boo-boo leg?" she asked.

"No, that's my better leg," I answered.

"I want you to have two better legs," she said.

"I am going to have two better legs soon," I promised.

She reached down and stroked my left thigh.

"But I can still walk," I said. "I just use crutches."

"I want a pair of crutches like Daddy's," she said. "You have to share."

I asked her if she wanted to go back to bed. She nodded. We walked the few steps to her door. Would she insist I come in? Would she start to cry? No. She padded off gleefully to bed and assumed her sleeping position. The magic had worked. The monsters were gone.

We have been touched, tickled, and just plain agog at the outpouring of best wishes. I've heard from half my high school class, a number of neighbors who remember

my bicycle accident as a boy, and nearly every girl I ever
kissed. I am heartsick at not being able to communicate
with each of you personally, but please know that
we are attacking this challenge with the full force of
determination, love, and humor. We find piercing shafts
of meaning on even the most challenging days. And we
treasure the reconnections this situation has spun.

Cancer, I have found, is a passport to intimacy. It's an
invitation—maybe even a mandate—to enter the most
vital, frightening, and sensitive human arenas. It's a
responsibility to address those issues we rarely want to
discuss, but we feel enriched when we do. In that spirit,
I hope you find occasion to ask a difficult question of
someone you love, renew a long-forgotten promise you
made to yourself, or spread a little magic of your own to
help keep the monsters at bay.

And, please, take a walk for me.

Love,

[signature]

· 8 ·

MAX

Pack Your Flip-Flops

IT BEGAN WITH A WALK. On the Saturday before classes began at Yale in 1983, huddles of freshmen gathered outside the dorms to trek together to the first football game of the season. One was a feisty schoolboy with hippy curly hair and cutoffs, who was so short and bookish he had been bullied in the Iowa town where he lived as a teenager, yet so smart and endearing his mother had trotted him out to beat her friends in chess. Another was me, preppier and a half a foot taller, but also fresh from growing up in a place where it was cooler to slay a rum and Coke than to read *To Kill a Mockingbird*.

We set out on the hour-long walk to the stadium and an hour later had spoken to no one else. What I remember most was the feeling—the absolute conviction—that this person would be in my life forever.

"Immediately I felt we were kindred souls," said Max, twenty-five years later. "Yet I tried to figure out where your self-awareness had come from. After all, unlike me, you hadn't lost your father when you were three. Your dad hadn't shot himself."

———

EVER SINCE THAT AFTERNOON, Max Stier was a constant presence in my life. Days might go by when we didn't talk; but, in a quarter century, a fortnight never passed when we didn't communicate. For two years we were roommates in college; for two months after our junior year we backpacked from Singapore to Beijing— getting stung by jellyfish in the Indian Ocean, urinating off the Great Wall, and getting booted from the lobbies of the great hotels because Max insisted on wearing tank tops and flip-flops.

That summer we made a pact to return to Asia when we were fifty, with whatever families we had, and stay in those hotels. Whichever one of us had made more money would have to foot the bill.

About halfway through that summer, Max and I arrived in northern Thailand. We arranged to go on an elephant safari with two blond backpackers from New Zealand. It had all the makings of a teenage male fantasy. But the night before, after we splurged on a meal of chicken, baby corn, and ice-cream sundaes, Max's stomach exploded and everything went running for the nearest exit. Soon he was splayed on the bathroom floor, covered in vomit, shaking. I did the only thing I could think to do: I doused him in water, wrapped him in a bedsheet, and carried him to the nearest hospital. Instead of spending the next three days riding elephants, smoking opium, and chasing my wet dreams, I was camped out in the emergency ward, in between Max and a dying man, whose family had built a Buddhist shrine in the corner.

Two decades later I was the one on the bathroom floor, heaving, shivering, and Max had flown in to be by my side, leaving his wife and two young sons at home. That's when I realized the grim bond we shared: Max's father had died when he was three, the same age as my girls. The man who knew me best had grown up in the situation I feared the most.

MAX STIER COMES FROM a family of fatherless sons. His maternal grandfather lost his father when he was thirteen and began pushing a fruit cart to support his family. Max's own father lost his father young. "My dad was an only child and my grandmother was extremely possessive of him," he said. "She was also very negative. I was on a kids' television show when I was six and was asked, 'Why does your grandmother love you?' I was supposed to give a cute answer, but I . . . didn't know the answer. That was the end of my television career."

"So what is the answer?" I asked.

"There is none. For someone like a grandparent or a parent, the answer is that they just do love you. It's the nature of the relationship. But the painful reality for me is that I've had very few of those relationships in my life."

Max's father, Herbert, was an orthopedic surgeon, a charmer, and a hard-driving father of three in the fall of 1969. "Apparently he was a very smart guy, overly ambitious, who wanted to succeed, so he pushed himself relentlessly," Max said. "He was doing research for the intellectual stimulation and consulting for the money. He started taking drugs to get up, to get down, to work, to sleep. He was trying to be Superman. Basically he had a psychotic break."

The housekeeper found him in the garage of their Tudor home in Los Angeles. He had a gun in his hand and a bullet hole in his heart. He left no note. Max's mother picked him up from nursery school and told him, "Your father is dead." When I met Max fourteen years later, he still believed the story his mother had told for all those years: The shooting had been an accident.

"She was waiting for us to ask," Max said. "And I think she was right. More dramatic for me is my complete lack of memory about the event—or my father. And when I think of my own kids, who are three and four now, I think, 'When do you cross that threshold when you maintain a conscious presence in your child?' I have no doubt I was impacted by my dad in ways I don't remember, but still, I can't remember."

"Do you have some keepsake?"

"I'm not a very materialistic person," he said. "I think I have a watch in a safety-deposit box somewhere. But truthfully, physical objects are not him for me. My connection is the stories I hear from people. My growing sense that he liked to kid around, that he was loyal and intellectually curious. All things I am."

I said one of the hard things for me is that my girls did not yet understand the meaning of death. "I met a woman recently who lost her husband," I said. "She told her eight-year-old daughter, 'Daddy is dead,' and her daughter said, 'Yes, I know. But when is he coming home?' Did you understand that your dad was dead?"

"When I was six, I had a series of nightmares," Max said. He paused to inhale. "This one is really hard to tell." His eyes reddened, and he squinched his nose in pain. His voice fell to a whisper. "The doorbell would ring and I'd get the door. And my dad would be there. But he'd look as if he'd just come out of the grave. Like a zombie. I didn't want to see him."

"What do you think those dreams meant?"

"I think it was part of my ambivalence," he said. "Part of me wanted him; part of me was afraid of him. And that tension was very strong."

"So let's just say that in ten years, Tybee and Eden come to you and say, 'You were the closest person to our father. The same thing happened to you that's happened to us. What do we do?'"

He reflected for a second.

"I would start by saying how much you loved them," Max said. "How I watched you blossom by having children. How good a dad you were. The most important thing a parent can do, I believe, is water a child profusely with love. I would water your children with love."

"What would you tell them to do with the pain?" I asked. "Should they confront it, or try to get over it?"

"It's not something you get over," he said. "It's something that's already a part of you. So you have to come at it directly—and keep coming back at it. The Jewish tradition of remembering those who have died every year is pretty useful. I cry once a year. I say the mourner's Kaddish and suddenly the emotion returns. I feel a deep hurt.

"But at the same," he said, "I would do something else. I would tell them stories. When you lose someone, the loss becomes the dominant memory. You have to build a rival memory. *We went here and did this. He took you there and did that.* By doing that, you help the girls find their own voice. They take the negative pain and create a positive side to it."

———

BEFORE SITTING DOWN TO speak with Max, I went back and read the journals I'd kept that summer we traveled together in Asia. Beside the youthful atrociousness of my own writing, what struck me most was how much hostility I felt toward him. Some of this antipathy probably came from my insecurities. Max was more confident and independent than I was at the time, and it bothered me. But part of this was his inflexibility. He had to have orange juice every morning before seven; he gave the Chinese lectures about customer service; he was fond of giving me discourses about how his Swiss Army knife could do more than mine.

May 30: "Max annoyed me a little bit today."
June 8: "I got really mad at Max tonight."
July 8: "Max is not the most sensitive friend I have."

At one point we actually split up for three days.

In retrospect, we were probably incompatible as roommates. Max is an early-to-bed, early-to-riser; I'm the opposite. Max insisted on doing push-ups and bench-pressing our backpacks every morning; I ate leftover dumplings. Max is obsessively neat; I'm only mostly neat. At one point we actually saw a production of *The Odd Couple* in Chinese.

But precisely because we endured those trials, our friendship became unbreakable. What happened in Shanghai stayed in Shanghai, and what was left was as enduring as the Great Wall. Max was my "Purple Heart," as in, "I went to war with this person, got wounded, but survived." He's the friend who nicked me a few times when we were younger, but our connection became so strong that the wounds soon melted away.

I would want him to tell the girls how we earned those wounds, of course—who we were when we first left home. But beyond that, I would want Max to embody for Eden and Tybee the values he has always represented to me. The loyalty of the friend who sees how far I've come instead of how far I have to go. The dignity of the person who has devoted his entire life to serving others. The self-respect of the man who insists on meeting his own standards instead of succumbing to those of others.

Max would teach them how to live.

"To me it all comes back to when I was a teenager being bullied in Iowa," Max said when I asked where those values came from. "I had to make a choice. I could change who I was and become more acceptable to the people around me, or I could stick to who I was and not worry about others. I decided that the world be damned, I was going to stick with who I was."

Armed with that self-reliance, Max became one of the most focused, efficient people I know. He was Phi Beta Kappa in college, clerked for the Supreme Court, counseled presidents. He started and still runs a nonprofit that encourages young people to go into public service. His confidence and sense of fairness were on display in one of the more selfless decisions Max ever made. He agreed to give his first son, Zachary, the surname of his wife, Florence Pan, the first Asian-American judge in the nation's capital.

"To me it was a no-brainer," Max explained. "There are no males in Florence's family, and it was meaningful for her dad to have the name continue. I honestly feel there is no legitimate reason why a child should have the father's name instead of the mother's. Plus, with our second son, we flipped. Noah got my name."

"You make it sound like a logic puzzle," I said.

"To me, it's part of equal parenting," he said. "When you're married to somebody, you need to put yourself in their shoes. There are some things I do better; some things Florence does better. But they have nothing to do with the particular XY chromosomes we have."

"Where does that attitude come from?"

"Part of it is a cultural norm," he said. "You're the same way. But there's no doubt that in my case it also comes from not having a dad myself. I value fatherhood more because I know what I lacked. And for me, the great thing about being a parent is that even though I feel like I didn't have much of a childhood as a boy, I'm having one now as a father."

As he talked I realized Max was speaking in a voice I had rarely heard him use. It was the voice of contentment. The fatherless boy had finally found peace in part by becoming a father himself. That morning, before coming to see me, he planted a vegetable garden with Zachary. That evening, he read a book to Noah on the phone and was genuinely worried about the golden treasure stolen by the pirates. That night, he was still wearing a tank top and flip-flops. Perhaps Max's greatest accomplishment is that he would still get kicked out of the great hotels of Asia for appearing too much like a child.

"So let's say we're lucky enough to make our trip when we're fifty," I said. "What will we have built in the intervening thirty years?"

"First of all, we're going to make it, Bu-ru-su," he said, using the Japanese version of my name. "And I think the answer is, we have a deeper love for each other. Part of it is sharing experiences over time, the encyclopedia of knowing someone forever. But the most important part is just being good friends. Someone who is there when you need help, there when you have something joyous to share, there to hold up a mirror so you can understand how you've changed."

"And are we going to stay in those fancy hotels?"

"Not if I have to wear long pants," he declared. "And not if I can't wear flip-flops."

"What's so important about flip-flops?"

"It's nothing to do with footwear," he said. "It's back to my philosophy of self-reliance over fitting in. I want to do the right thing, and to me that means not wearing too much clothing in a tropical sweatbox."

As soon as he said that, I suddenly flashed to that kid in curly hair and cutoffs I first met when we were teen-agers—bookish, boyish, ready to outsmart you in chess, and able to turn his defiant taste in shoes into an endur-ing axiom of personal integrity: No matter where you are, you should always be true to yourself. No matter where you go, you should always pack your flip-flops.

9

THE LESSON OF THE DUNES

W HEN PEOPLE HEAR THAT I am a writer, they often ask if I learned it from my dad. "My dad never wrote anything longer than a memo," I usually quip.

But what memos!

My father is the master of the memo pad. The Shakespeare of sticky notes. Few people I know say more with less.

From the time we were kids, we got stacks of news articles slipped under our doors (later they were faxed, then e-mailed, now texted), each with a specific coding: *R&R* meant read and return; a double arrow meant read and pass along to the next person. We got reams of note-paper encrypted with his paternal haiku.

> *Your will / Let's discuss / When?*
> *Cleaning the porch / Sunday morning /*
> *Command performance.*

These dispatches were invariably written in flat-line cursive with blue, red, or green felt-tip ink. And they would never be longer than ten words. On the day of a piece of bad news: *How do we solve the problem?* On the morning of a big transition: *Don't look back.*

My dad makes Twitter seem expansive.

When he turned sixty, we gathered a number of my father's most memorable Dad-isms and put them in a book.

> *If you don't like it, don't eat it, but don't kick.*
> *If it can be solved with time or money,*
> *it's not a problem.*
> *As long as you're still talking, you're still negotiating.*

Some were wicked, like his comment whenever a child took a tumble: *Did you hurt the floor?* Some were wise, like his remark about his mother's Alzheimer's: *It's more difficult to bring down parents than to bring up kids.*

At least three are enduring. They grew out of the pivotal moments in my upbringing and became the proverbs that most embody my father to me.

———

MY DAD IS ONE of those men who become better-looking

the older they get. The distinguished seventy-year-old with the bald pate and silver temples who reminds people of Gene Hackman was once a skinny Eagle Scout with nerd-wavy hair and Dumbo ears. Edwin Feiler Jr. was an awkward child, and he was often overshadowed by his dashing younger brother, Stanley. When their father built a subdivision, he named the prized front street after Stanley, the rear one after my dad.

"Stanley was just more polished," my father said. "When I was fifteen, my father took us to Hunter Army Airfield and tried to teach me how to drive. He failed. Yet Stanley, who was only twelve, picked it up. He was just easier to train. He was always popular. He had better social skills. You could take him places where I wouldn't fit in."

What my father had was discipline and determination. Those rabbit ears aside, he was the classic tortoise. He gritted his way into the top ten of his class at the Savannah High School, the Wharton School at the University of Pennsylvania, and navy ROTC. When I asked him how he became an Eagle Scout, he said, simply: "I try to complete the things I start."

Ironically, a rare lapse in that self-control became a central moment in his life. He called it "the hour that changed my life." "In 1956 I was commissioned into the navy and sent to training school," he said. "My grades gave me the right to pick any assignment, and I chose to be stationed in Europe. But several weeks before graduation, I cut a cooking class and took a nap. I thought I wouldn't get caught, and I got caught. That's how I got assigned to the U.S.S. *Wisconsin* in Norfolk, Virginia, which is how I ended up marrying your mother."

"So your delinquency brought us here today!"

"Absolutely. And I was not normally a very delinquent guy."

Two years later, on the day my mother was supposed to attend her graduation from the University of Michigan, Edwin Feiler and Jane Abeshouse were married in Baltimore. Her mother serenaded them with a homespun version of "Dixie."

> They're on their way to the land of cotton
> Ed and Jane won't be forgotten . . .
> In Dixie-Land they'll be so happy
> Grits and juleps to keep them snappy

The next year they moved back to Savannah and settled into my great-grandmother's old house. "When I left Savannah in 1952, I thought I would never come back," my father said. "Savannah wasn't much of a place. There was no air-conditioning. No television. The only people who had TV set up giant antennae to receive one or two stations from Jacksonville. There were tons of unpaved streets, even downtown. Lady Astor said Savannah was like a beautiful woman with a dirty face. She was right! Plus, it was highly and uncomfortably segregated."

But something changed along the way. He did. "When I was living in the Northeast, I realized I didn't like the values of the New York–New Jersey corridor," my father said. "One night in college, I was in the Bryn Mawr train station after taking out this girl, and I said to myself, 'I don't want to live here. Savannah's a much better place to raise children.'"

The gambit paid off. By the 1960s, Savannah was on the move, my father was finding success building houses, and my mother was pregnant. But when my brother was born in October 1961, crisis. The eight-pound, eight-ounce baby had an enormous growth protruding from the bottom of his spine, a rare defect called a myelo-meningocele. "It was this big blob, sticking out of his body, that was larger than his head," my father recalled.

My mom's father, Bucky, a prominent urologist, was in the delivery room. "When Bucky saw it, the first thing he did was scratch the instep of the baby's foot," my dad said. "Andy wiggled his toes. Bucky concluded that the boy's spinal cord was intact and said that even though only one in ten thousand people with this birth defect ever walked, Andy could be the one." The next day a team of thirteen doctors removed the growth and closed my brother's spine. After the surgery, Bucky assured my mother that her son would live a normal life and said he had to return to Baltimore to operate.

A month later Bucky Abeshouse had a heart attack and died.

"Since that time," my father said, "whenever I hear that somebody had a baby, I always say, 'Is it healthy?' because in twenty-four hours the responsibilities of fatherhood came down on me very, very quickly."

For two years, doctors measured my brother's head every other month to make sure he was developing normally. After learning that he was, my parents consulted with experts at Emory University as to whether they should have more children. The doctors saw no reason not to try.

"When Dr. Bodziner came out of the delivery room on October 25, 1964," my father said, "the first thing he said to me was that you were healthy. That was a huge relief. Because remember, only one in ten thousand with that condition ever walk, and we'd already had the one."

———

WHENEVER I CONJURE UP images of my father from my childhood, he's usually sitting down: at the head of the dinner table carving a roast; in the living room smoking a pipe; on the beach reading a novel. I have strong memories of him coming into my bedroom every night when I was in high school, pulling up a chair, and asking if I had anything to talk about. I usually brushed him off and went back to my homework, but the message was clear that he was open for counsel.

He was certainly active—played badminton, was an early jogger, took walks—but the values he conveyed were thronelike: wisdom, stability, calmness. He was, in the best sense of the word, settled.

And when I think of the wisdom he passed on from his seat of power, three pearls stand out.

The first occurred when I was thirteen. It was the night of my bar mitzvah, and my parents had invited friends over to our house. Near the end of the party, my father called me over to the bar, ordered a gin and tonic, and handed it to me. "You're a man now," he said. "You're responsible for your own actions." And if I ever had too much to drink, he said, it would be among the greatest pleasures of his life if I would call him and ask him to come pick me up.

The moment was classic Ed Feiler: trusting, indirectly emotional, constantly nudging us out of the nest. It was his way of saying, as he often did, that he was our cheerleader. His goal was to provide the shoulders on which we would climb into the sky. He wanted nothing more than to be "between the commas" in some magazine, as in "Bruce Feiler, son of Mr. and Mrs. Edwin J. Feiler, reached some milestone this week."

I didn't fully realize what he was trying to say until I, too, became a parent. The higher joy is not the light, it's the reflection. The greater pleasure is not climbing up; it's handing down.

Between the commas

THE SECOND OCCURRED WHEN I was seventeen. I was co–vice president of my junior class, and our chief responsibility was to throw the prom. A month before the date, we lost our venue. A deal was swiftly done to move the prom to the Savannah Yacht Club, but it discriminated against blacks and Jews. In a fit of uncharacteristic bravado, my fellow VP, Laura, and I objected. Our car-wash and bake-sale bounty would not feed their coffers.

As soon as we complained, my parents sat us down. "It's time you learned about Charlie Wittenstein," they said. An attorney and veteran of discrimination battles, Charlie had three rules for such situations.

1. *Keep your cool.*
2. *Never threaten.* The other side will believe you are much more powerful than you really are.
3. *Give them a graceful out.* Even though you may prevail, let them believe you didn't get everything you wanted.

Forever after we called them the Charlie Wittenstein Rules.

"And let me tell you," my father said later. "They really, really work."

That afternoon, in an attempt to provide a "graceful out," Laura and I identified a dozen alternate venues. The school called a board meeting, and my mother went as our spokesperson. A community college was chosen as the final venue. After the meeting, our class mother approached my mom. "Congratulations, Jane," she said, syrup in her voice. "By the way, how would you like to be chair of the decorating committee?"

Our comeuppance was getting up at 6 A.M. on prom morning to hang crepe paper fish from the rafters.

———

THE FINAL LESSON TOOK place when I was twenty-three. In 1988, after spending a year teaching English in Japan, I returned to Savannah. I had been writing you-can't-believe-what-happened-to-me letters home, and now everywhere I went, people said to me, "I love your letters." I looked at them. "Have we met?" My grandmother had been photocopying the letters and passing them around. I had an idea, "Maybe I should write a book."

I was twenty-three years old. I didn't know anyone who had written a book. I didn't know anything about the book business. But I had a secret weapon. I had my dad. During a talk on the beach, he urged me to take the leap.

"I'll tell you the same thing I told your brother when he was trying to decide whether to move to England for a year," he said. "Take a year. Give it a try. When you're fifty years old, you will have spent two percent of your life trying to make your dream come true. And when you look back, I think you'll realize it was a good two percent."

The Two Percent Rule

Few things in my life have proven to be so 100 percent correct.

———

SOME MONTHS INTO MY cancer treatment, Linda and I received a rare letter from my father. It began:

Dear Bruce and Linda,

The United States Navy released me from active duty on March 29, 1959. I had the benefit of a great education and visited a lot of the world, yet I wanted to live in Savannah because it was the best place I had seen to raise a family. My energetic and loving wife agreed. We drove our new, un-air-conditioned Chevrolet (cost $2,181) from Annapolis to Savannah. I immediately went to work for Metro Developers. My first day on the job was Wednesday, April 1, 1959, and I am still here.

In fifty years I have had one job, one city and one wife.

My father went through twenty drafts of this letter, he explained, which he sent to all his children. It was inspired by a lunch at the Commerce Club in Atlanta, in which a friend asked how he was, and my father answered, "I have three children, all of whom get along well with one another, understand the value of money, and have the work ethic. Everything else is in second place."

His friend replied, "I know everybody in this room, and no one else can make that statement."

The letter went on to tout his Family First philosophy, which had defined my father through three recessions, four grandchildren, two hurricanes, and one osteosarcoma. "We intend to continue this philosophy," he wrote.

Later I asked him where he would take his grandchildren to pass along this philosophy. "I would take them to the dunes of Tybee," he said. "And I would explain that when I first started walking here forty years ago, these dunes were only pimples. Today, they are mountainous, with grass and sea oats, and pines.

"And the lesson of the dunes," he continued, "is that you are a part of a continuum. Change occurs over a long period of time. So don't be in a hurry. Recognize your limitations. But know that if you reach back in history and understand how you got here, you will be more prepared for the future."

His letter to us ended:

I am not going anywhere for a while (I hope) because our work together is so enjoyable and productive. Please accept my personal thanks for being such an effective part of our team.

It was signed, in a way his father would have rec-
ognized, "With great affection, Edwin J. Feiler, Jr." But
then, in a touch of grace that showed he had learned from
the missteps of the previous generation, he had crossed
off the typewritten valediction, and scribbled in two
words in blue felt-tip ink.

Love, Dad

10

CHRONICLES OF THE LOST YEAR

volume III

October 1

Dear Friends and Family,

Even as summer drifted from view, September was the
most beautiful month we have seen for some time in
Brooklyn, with bright skies, clear nights, and just a hint
of coolness in the air. We are beginning to get whiffs of
fall and the outbreak of pumpkins and spray-on cobwebs
that mark the arrival of Halloween, a national holiday in
kid-friendly Brooklyn Heights.

A few weeks ago my parents and in-laws arrived to
help celebrate Linda's significant birthday. ("Mommy's
turning forty!" Tybee announced to everyone who would
listen.) The day corresponded with the beginning of

round three of my chemotherapy. I stayed in bed all day so I could rouse enough energy to sit upright for a few hours that night in a restaurant. After the meal I crutched my way to the bathroom and asked the waiter to stick a candle in a chocolate cake for Linda. When the cake arrived with no candle, I nearly lunged at the man, who apologized and returned moments later with a solo scoop of lemon verbena sorbet with a single candle perched on top. Linda held her breath and prepared to blow, and for the first time I can ever remember, none of us wondered what she was wishing for.

We were all wishing for the same thing.

Three months have passed since I first learned I have bone cancer, and our lives for the moment have settled into a new normal. I have been through three of the four rounds of Cisplatin and Adriamycin I am slated to get before the surgery. While each time I get knocked out for about ten days, we have all somehow managed to adjust to the discomfort, exhaustion, and dislocation. The early signs suggest these treatments may be having a positive effect. My tumor has shrunk by about one-third; some of the warning levels in my blood have returned to near normal; I have more mobility. As my otherwise circumspect oncologist reported, "You're kicking this tumor's butt." And my surgeon observed, "Only green flags, no yellow or red."

Having said that, both of my doctors have prepared me for the reality that my body will probably not bounce back quite as well from future treatments, that a host of complications still linger at every turn, and that the surgery itself will take quite a toll. But in the meantime, they are happily adding a third, more toxic drug to my regimen. This month I will begin four rounds of high-dose Methotrexate. (Query: Why do chemo drugs all have names that sound like comic book villains? *Now that the evil, octo-armed Cisplatin has been felled, here comes the dastardly Methotrexate to threaten Gotham City. . . .*) Methotrexate is given in weekly doses, not triweekly, so we're bracing for a relentless few months in advance of the surgery.

So what's it like around there? A challenge. I'm skinnier than at any time since our wedding. I'm bald. I'm on crutches. A cold I caught this week lasted three times longer than it normally would have. Just the other night I lay awake in bed, muttering to myself, "Nothing good ever happens to me anymore." Later, I had a dream in which I imagined life around my home after I had died and was no longer living here. It ended with me walking into my office and seeing photos of someone else's children on my desk. I screamed a deep-throated scream and woke up.

We have been struck that our situation raises one unfamiliar challenge. We are at an age when many of our friends are dealing with the issues surrounding aging parents. As unpleasant as these issues are, most of us know we will face them—and know many who already have. But when the person getting sick has four living parents, as I do (counting mine and my in-laws), the illness overturns the natural order of life. Few of us have the emotional vocabulary to deal with this reality, especially when those parents move back in for a while.

More than once I have scowled at my mother for treating me like a child or suddenly prying too deeply into my bowel movements or sex life. (No, I didn't check whether Cisplatin could be countervailed by Viagra, but thanks for asking.) I growled when my mother-in-law called an air-conditioning repairman for our guestroom, when the device just wasn't turned on. If nothing else, we need our parents now, and we are grateful for the disruption they are causing to their own lives to help us—and our daughters—thrive. But setting new rules has been trying.

As for Linda, her life can be pretty crummy these days— from daily insurance battles to a perpetual slog through hospital waiting rooms to a husband who barely looks up from his pillow. I spend a lot of time staring into space. Linda keeps saying, "I'm so sorry this is happening to you" or "You don't deserve this," but I don't often find it comforting. One night recently I was performing my grim bedtime ritual: putting down my crutches, pulling my pants and underwear down to my ankles, sitting down gingerly on the bed, pulling my pants and underwear up over my right foot, then, after lifting my left leg carefully with two hands, kicking them off my left. I then repeat the entire exercise in reverse with my pajamas, a humiliating routine that has now added nearly a full minute of stomach-wrenching indignity to the simplest of everyday tasks.

Observing the look on my face, Linda asked, innocently, caringly, "What's wrong?"

"My life sucks, that's what's wrong," I snapped. I instantly felt miserable. I took her in my arms and kissed her. "I'm ruining your life," I said. "I feel so bad."

Even with all this agony, Linda managed to find some joy in recent weeks. She helped our girls have a wonderful summer, including time with the Rottenbergs on Cape Cod and the Feilers on Tybee Island. Her friends showered her with cupcakes and massages for her birthday. And though it will be taxing on us, I am excited that Linda is scheduled to make brief trips to California, Argentina, and Dubai in the coming months.

The girls, meanwhile, are doing great. A few blips aside, Tybee and Eden are sprouting with maturity and showing fewer signs of stress. They were gleeful at learning to swim by themselves at the beach this August. They daily prance around, belting out their new theme song, from *The Sound of Music:* "I am sixteen going on seventeen," including the gem that they are completely unprepared "to face a world of men." And they are so consumed by reading that they regularly correct our spelling.

We had a moment of crisis a few weeks back when during a regularly scheduled tea party, a friend asked our darling Purplicious (Eden) and Pinkalicious (Tybee) what their favorite colors were. Eden, per years of preference, said "purple and rainbow." Then Tybee, overturning equal years of pink intransigence, also said "purple and rainbow." For a second time stopped, the heavens parted, and it was one of those moments as in the Book of Joshua when God seemed on the verge of hurling the planets toward Earth. We all felt as if we were witnessing a once-in-a-lifetime alteration, like the changing of the Coke formula or the fall of the Berlin Wall. Linda was ready to cheer this sign of growing up, but Daddy quickly stepped in. "Mommy has already bought you a college tuition's worth of pink sweaters, coats, mittens, and snowsuits. I'll be darned if you'll wear *anything but pink* until spring." The Old World Order was quickly restored.

So what's the big picture? After months of living with cancer, I still find it easier to be at home rather than venture too far into the world. Here everybody knows I'm sick, and it's safer. Often when I'm driving down a busy street and looking out at all the pedestrians, I think to myself,

"That person doesn't have cancer. That person doesn't either." Seeing other people walk without thinking can bring on a surge of sadness—or anger. "Do you know how lucky you are?!" I want to shout. As someone said to me recently, "We all have a gun pointing at our heads; it's just easy to forget." This year, at least, we won't forget.

Still, the many e-mails, letters, and gestures we have received from far and wide have reminded us that we are not alone, and that even as we all hurry down the avenues of our own lives, there are many invisible eyes looking out for us and prepared to hurl a few planets our way if the need arises.

Thank you for being a part of that, and if these letters have caused you to pause even for a few minutes in a busy day, perhaps you'll consider some of the gestures that have brought meaning to our family. Write a Friday missive to a forgotten friend. Reach out to someone you kissed—or kissed off—long ago. Remember a forgotten wish.

Or, take a walk for me.

Love,

Bruce

11

DAVID

Don't See the Wall

THE FIRST TIME I MET David Black he was sitting in a blue velour barrel chair in his office overlooking the Flatiron Building on Fifth Avenue in Manhattan. Five foot three and a half, on a good day, in cowboy boots, he rubbed his fingers together like a shaman and peered out eagerly, like a mongoose ready to pounce, managing to be both cute and fierce, lovable but still capable of killing a cobra.

Six years into my writing career, I had hit a wall. I had three books published but had no visible path to earning a living. In a final act of desperation, I left my mother-knows-best agent and went looking for help. With a platoon of bestseller lists on his wall and a roster of rising stars he helped manage, David Black was recommended as a would-be savior. A sports fan and work-out fiend, David also had something none of the other candidates on my list had: a penis.

He soon started proving it. He took one look at my six-foot-two body and announced, even before I sat down, "If I were your height I'd be in the NBA."

Self-delusion is a beautiful thing, but bravado is even better.

Especially in an agent.

Within days he was peppering me with phone calls and telling me that my entire approach to fulfilling my dreams was wrong. To a dreamer flat against the bricks of disappointment, the words were magic. I signed on eagerly.

But still I wondered: How do I get over the wall?

———

ONE UNEXPECTED GIFT OF the Council of Dads was that it forced me to formalize what otherwise would have gone unsaid. It obliged me to sit down with my closest friends, tell them what they meant to me, then ask them to play an important role for my daughters. As my treatment ticked on and the surgery grew closer, the men in my Council would have been there already. The daily postcards from Jeff were gathering by my bed; Max's fortnightly phone calls grew to three times a week. But by inviting these men into the innermost space of our lives, we were cementing a new kind of bond.

And by forcing us to sit down and discuss our lives, I began to detect certain patterns among these men. First was a new kind of maleness, one that would have been completely alien to my father's father, or even to my own father, who has a more distant relationship with even his oldest male friends. For starters, we talk—and fairly regularly. More important, we talk about things that were once the exclusive domain of women's magazines and daytime chat shows: our children, our feelings, even our bodies.

For me, no friend represents this new vernacular of modern manhood more than David Black. David is both a classic man's man and a modern woman's man. On the manly front, he picks up the phone with "Yo, motherfucker!" He's hypercompetitive and prone to giving endless paeans about obscure bottles of wine. He even bought a convertible sports car for his fiftieth birthday. (Actually, like many a true guy, he's impatient: He bought it on his forty-ninth.)

On the new-man front, he leaves work early to coach Little League, he hugs, he's the first person to call when distress breaks and the last one to check in at the end of a crummy day. And he bakes. Someone asked me if David cried when I invited him to join my Council of Dads. "David cries when you invite him for a walk," I said.

Part of this personality mix comes from deep childhood insecurities about his size and weight. I asked him what he looked like when he was younger. "I was chunky as a kid," he said. "What does *chunky* mean?" I asked. His answer came swift. "Fat."

David was born in Jackson Heights, Queens. His father was an editor at William Morrow, and the first book he published was Reginald Damerell's *Triumph in a White Suburb: The Dramatic Story of Teaneck, N.J., the First Town in the Nation to Vote for Integrated Schools.* Hillel Black was so besotted with this bedroom community that he relocated his family there when David was eight.

"Because my father was an editor, he used to work from home on Fridays," David said. "I would always ask him to come out and play, and he wouldn't because he had to work. He would sit alongside one of those old tube radios, listening to opera. I grew up hating opera because he would never come and play. To this day, I don't like opera."

Did he romanticize books because of his father?

"I admired what my father did, but I never wanted to do it. I wanted to work for myself. When I was a kid, I wanted a stereo. My parents told me I could have one, but only if I earned the money to pay for it. So I got a paper route. I delivered the *Bergen Record* off the back of my bicycle. After a few weeks, my mother drove by in the car and said, 'Your father and I have been talking, and we've decided we'll buy you a stereo.' I said, 'Mom, you can keep driving. I have a paper route to do.' "

David's self-reliance, which at times can be bullheadedness, became a hallmark of his personality. At twenty-one, he finally applied it to the one arena that most plagued him as a child. "I was working at Macy's," David said, "and I had put on a lot of weight. So I started running. From April to October I dropped forty pounds and entered the New York City marathon. It was the single most formative experience of my life. Hands down. Not even close. Because it taught me that I can do what I set out to do. It harkened back to that time delivering newspapers. I had a goal. I was going to realize that goal. And nothing was going to stand in my way."

Not even his father.

"I ran the last half of the race half an hour faster than the first," David said. "And as I came to the twenty-fifth mile, my father came out into the road, happy to see me. I looked up and said, 'Fuck off.' I felt terrible the moment I said it, but I realized what I was doing. This was my moment. Nobody was going to take it from me. It's no accident that a week later I met my wife."

"You credit the marathon with meeting Melissa?" I asked.

"I was feeling good about myself. I was ready. Most men don't articulate concerns about their bodies, but I bet you most men think about them. How often do you see somebody in the street with his belly hanging out over his belt, and he walks with a sense of anger about himself? You don't feel good about yourself, you're not going to be happy. I would tell that to your girls."

———

ONE HALLMARK OF THIS new breed of men is that the old boundaries of male bonding no longer apply. David is the colleague who also became a friend; now he's the friend who's also a colleague. No one on my Council of Dads knows my work life better than David; and, because he lives nearby, few know my home life better. Our families have a regular calendar of Halloween trick-or-treat visits, Super Bowl parties, birthday celebrations. (David and I share a birthday, though, ahem, he shared it alone for five years before me.)

There are advantages to this kind of relationship: a seamlessness between work and family, a comfort that the people who help you make professional decisions understand the consequences for your personal life. But there are drawbacks, too: It's harder to get away, and, if things go wrong, it's harder to extricate yourself. I've experienced both sides with David.

A literary agent is a broker of dreams in a world in which most dreams don't come true. It's this aspect of David—his finesse at handling aspirations *and* setbacks—that is his greatest skill, and the gift Linda and I most wanted him to share with our daughters. David would push the girls to imagine some unimaginable goal, then pick themselves up when that goal proved elusive.

David would teach them how to dream.

David Black began his career in the book business

delivering mail in a large New York agency. He moved on to answer phones at another, then finally got the courage to start his own. He was twenty-nine years old. "When I was a kid, I was walking with my father on our front lawn one day, and he said to me, 'Son, I don't really care what you do in life. Own it.' That stuck with me, and the day I incorporated, I called my dad. 'There are one hundred shares in Black Inc.,' I said, 'and you are talking to the man who owns all of them.'"

"Were you scared?"

"I was never scared until I signed my first payroll check. That's when I realized that somebody else's family was eating in part because of the work that I was doing."

"When did you know it would work?"

He didn't blink. "I never thought it wouldn't."

David has certain assets that make him good at his job. He thinks schematically and is somewhat impatient, which helps him find structure in often disjointed book ideas. When I wanted to follow five country music artists in Nashville for a year, he persuaded me to cut it to three. He was right. He's entrepreneurial yet sensitive to corporate culture, which helps him craft creative deals. When I wanted to publish a book of photographs from my travels in the Middle East—a quixotic and surely money-losing idea—he suggested that my publisher and I share the costs, thereby splitting the risk and any upside. The book was published successfully.

But most of all he's emotional, with well-plumbed insecurities of his own, which helps him manage the emotional sinkholes and bottomless insecurities of his clients. A year after our initial meeting, when David tried to sell my fourth book, he blundered the auction, and overnight I'd lost a year's income. It was devastating for me, yet somehow worse for him. "The most humiliating experience of my career," he still calls it. As I stood face-to-face with another professional roadblock, David flew halfway across the country, slept on my couch, and vowed to walk by my side. It was a mutual treaty of neediness.

"That's why I cried on the day you made the bestseller list," David said.

Seven years later, at the bottom of my life, the day Linda and I had our first meeting with Dr. Healey, David came to our home to slip on my shoes, shoulder my bag, and watch my back as I teetered down the stairs, into the taxi, up to the waiting room, and into the void of unknowing.

Later, after the tears and the fear, after the poison started ravaging my blood, after I'd stopped writing altogether, I asked David what he learned from all these years as a curator of dreams. What's the most important gift you can give to a dreamer?

"The belief in their ability to succeed," he said without pause. "Because when you believe in them, you give them the strength to believe in themselves."

"But at that moment when I first walked into your office," I said, "I didn't believe. I'd been working my dream for a decade, and I wasn't making it. I was at a wall."

"I don't see the wall," he said. "And I'm telling you to be the same way. 'Don't see the wall.' Of course you may encounter a wall from time to time, but you tear it down, walk through it. You find a way to get over it, or around it, or under it. You acknowledge it but move beyond it. Whatever you do, don't succumb to it. Don't give in to the wall."

"So it's twenty years from now," I said. "Tybee or Eden Feiler plops down in your barrel chair. She has a dream. She wants to open a restaurant, or climb a mountain, or run a marathon, or write a book. But she's scared. *I can't. It's too hard. I don't have the money.* What do you tell her?"

"I tell her, 'Let's sit down and figure out what's possible,'" he said. "'Let's make a road map to the top of the mountain, or a business plan for the restaurant, or an outline for the book. Let's make the awesome mundane.'"

At times like this, David's voice loses its bravado and its bluster. It gives up its towel-snapping manliness altogether. It shrinks instead to a near whisper and swells with the empathy of that chunky little boy, alone in the backyard, just waiting for the opera to end, who knows what it's like to not believe in yourself and to want what you cannot have.

"And if, for some reason, that dream should fail?" I asked.

"Then I tell her, 'Let's find a dream that can work,'" he said. "It may not be the first dream, or the dream of the moment. But you shift your dreams. You find a dream that might come true. And when it does, you focus on the joy of the success rather than the devastation of defeat. Because in my experience, anybody can dream an impossible dream. But only a few find a dream that's possible.

"And those are the ones that are happy."

12

USE YOUR WORDS

Long before I had cancer, I had a secret game I played with myself involving my kids. It was a memory exercise. A way of cheating time. Basically it was an errand into the impossible: I tried to guess what they would remember.

We would be biking through the dunes, or planting flowers in the backyard, or dripping turrets onto sand castles, and they would be having the perfect reaction. They would be happy, or ignited by a new idea, or simply free of the gossamer of complications that ensnares childhood. And I would say to myself: *This is the moment they will always remember. This is the experience that will mark this age forever.*

When I got sick, this game took on new urgency.

Friends tried to comfort me: "Don't worry. Your children are so young, your illness will become a distant memory for them. After all, how many memories do you have from when you were three?" These comments were anything but comforting: If my children remembered little from these years, that meant, if I died, they would remember little of me.

Even more unnerving, now that I had trouble walking, we were restricted in the types of memories we could build. Left without legs, I fell back on their one true passion. I turned to words.

One day a few months into my treatment, I invited Tybee and Eden into my bed. "How about a reading party?" I said. They squealed and returned with armfuls of their favorite books: *Angelina Ballerina, The Jellybeans and the Big Dance, Thesaurus Rex.* For an hour we were a dad's fantasy of a living library—all giggles, dramatic accents, concerned expressions, and throaty cheers. These weren't books as babysitters. These were books as bridges.

Somewhere in the middle, I closed a book and announced, "Girls, I want to tell you something." My voice got all drippy and earnest. "If you always read books, you'll always be happy." They nodded, repeated what I'd said, then returned to their books.

Suddenly that feeling came over me: *This is it,* I thought. *This is the phrase they'll never forget. This is the one story they'll tell their first boyfriends when they're lying on the quadrangle and recounting their life stories.*

I started choking up. A day with cancer is a day with tears. But playtime was coming to an end, so I managed to wrangle their attention once more. "Thank you for Daddy time," I said. "And remember . . ."

I looked at them, hoping they would repeat my line. I wanted them to tell me we had been communicating. I wanted them to reassure me they'd always remember who I was.

"If you always read books . . . ," I said, and it was Tybee who answered. "You'll always be smart."

Well, yes!

I laughed out loud.

WE WERE OVERWHELMED FIRST-TIME parents in the early hours after the girls were born. The initial days were a swirl of blockaded milk ducts, nonlatching mouths, and landfills of diapers. The biggest challenge we faced was not the lack of sleep or backlogged belches but the Olympian gymnastics of breast-feeding two newborns simultaneously. Linda could either feed them serially, which meant she was back on virtual bed rest, or use the "double football," in which she clasped a baby under each arm like an overeager running back. Neither worked very well. The upshot was we starved one and dropped the other in the first week. Our doctor was growing concerned about our fecklessness.

Eventually we settled into an awkward pose, in which a feeding involved three adults. Linda provided the *mise en place;* one adult held up one baby, and someone else held up the other. We kept an elaborate spreadsheet chronicling who had eaten what, drank how much supplement, peed what amount, and pooped what volume. Some weeks into this routine, I was recounting this tale of survival to a table of friends and mentioned how hard we had been working to breast-feed our daughters. *"We??"* a mom friend sternly corrected. "You mean *she*!!!"

"No," I insisted, staking a flag for forgotten dads, "I mean we!!"

Then I relayed my martyr's tale of kneeling outside the passenger's door of our station wagon during a recent outing, thundershowers pummeling my back, as I lifted one of my daughters like a burnt offering to God so she could suckle on Linda's nipple. "The first time one of my girls says she hates her father," I announced, "I'm going to re-create this pose!"

(For the record, none of the other moms was impressed.)

Once we figured out how to keep the girls alive, we could finally think about their development. And from the beginning, we were nervous about words. The most common question we were asked as parents of twins was, "Do they have their own language?" Twin talk, or idioglossia, is a condition in which twins develop a private language incomprehensible to outsiders. The principal explanation, we were told, is that children learn to speak by mimicking those around them, and twins spend more time staring at each other than at their parents. Also, grown-ups rarely speak to twins face-to-face, more often addressing them as a pair.

Enunciation became our obsession. Phonics was our focus. Forget stage parents: We were diphthong parents. And whether it was genetics or overcompensation, the process worked. Our girls talked before they walked; they knew their ABCs by a year; by eighteen months they were losing themselves in menus and catalogs; and by two and a half they were reciting Dr. Seuss in the accent of Mary Poppins. "Use your words," we begged when they threw tantrums, but more often we pleaded for the opposite. "Stop talking and go to sleep!" Idioglossia who? Our girls loved to talk.

Except when others were around. When the doorbell rang, our nonstop chatterers suddenly turned into ardent mimes. To circumvent their shyness, we devised a list of questions for them to grill every visitor: When is your birthday? What did you have for breakfast? What is your favorite place? Eventually they added a question of their own—What is your favorite Disney princess?—and that's when we knew it was time for another game.

We called it "Reporters." Killing time one day in an airport, I sent the girls to far-flung corners to count the number of seats, ascertain the color of a sign, or ask a jet-lagged passenger where she lived. Each girl was charged with announcing her name and giving a report on her findings.

But the most effective tool we found for building meaning through words was a game I played every night as a child: Bad & Good. Dinner was sacred in my house. My siblings and I were encouraged to do our own activities in the afternoons, but 6:00 P.M. dinner was untouchable. Every night we followed the same routine. A designated moderator would go around the table and ask each person, "What happened bad to you today?" My parents offered bads, too, and the effect was to show their vulnerabilities in a sort of real-time tutorial in coping with disappointments. The one hard-and-fast decree: "You can't knock someone else's bad."

The next round of questions was upbeat. "What happened good to you today?" The value of ending with positives was lost on none of us, but the game has an irresistible structure and intimacy.

When Linda and I initiated Bad & Good with the girls, they didn't grasp the rules at first. They would repeat *our* bads—"I didn't get enough sleep"—or mimic each other's—"Mine is the same as hers." But in time they grew more confident in expressing their feelings: "My sister stole my tiara" or "Mommy stayed with us all day!" The game became a way to chart their individuation. It also helped show that difficult conversations can be had with people of all ages, often with conflicting points of view—as long as you learn not to knock them.

THIS MADE IT ALL the more surprising when we didn't follow our own advice.

As I accumulated more rounds of chemotherapy through the fall, my body began to deteriorate. I shed weight like tears; my immune system grew weaker; my eyebrows and eyelashes tumbled with the leaves. More disturbing, I was hospitalized repeatedly. These five-day confinements would come on suddenly. In the morning I would be uncomfortable, but fine; by the afternoon my fever would spike to 103.5, and I was forced to hurry to Urgent Care. My white and red blood counts would flat-line, leaving me vulnerable to colds, flus, pneumonias, and most of the other contagions preschoolers routinely bring home. I caught every one. We bought facial masks in bulk.

But the most significant decision we made was not to tell the girls where I was going. To be fair, this had been mostly my decision. The girls didn't know what a hospital was, and I didn't want to concern them.

It was a huge mistake.

In early November I returned from a five-day stint on the twelfth floor at Memorial Sloan-Kettering Hospital and resumed my bedtime duties with the girls. In recent months I had been playing a game in which I asked each of them to say two things she wanted to hear in a story, and I would then weave them into a fairy tale. I liked this game because it was a high-wire act every night and taught me more about storytelling than any graduate seminar. The girls liked it because they got to participate. Tybee usually insisted on something pink; Eden invariably requested two girls in dresses.

On my first night home from the hospital, I asked them what they wanted in their story. Tybee: "A pink frog and strawberry ice cream." Eden: "Two girls who don't have a family."

Uh-oh.

The next morning, after Eden erupted into a meltdown, I led her to the crying chair. "Why did you request two girls who don't have a family?" I asked. "Do *you* have a family?"

"Yes."

"Who?"

She pointed to me, then added, "Mommy and Tybee."

"Are you scared sometimes that you don't have a family?"

She nodded. "When you and Mommy go away from the house."

I almost didn't want to ask the next question. "Were you scared when Daddy went away this weekend?"

"I was very, very, very, very scared," Eden said.

That's four *verys*.

My heart sank. That afternoon we got a call from the teachers. "The girls are being a little clingy these days, is something going on around the house?" That night I introduced a new game. It was called: "Would you like to ask Daddy a question?"

Eden went first. I brought her into my office and carefully explained that Daddy went to the hospital during his trips away from home, and that the doctors took care of him there. Did she have any questions about the hospital?

"Where do you sleep?" she said. I explained that they have beds. "Does it hurt?" No.

When her turn came, Tybee was more probing. "What do they do with the red parts under your skin?" "How do they see inside you?" "When they stick a hole in you, how do they close you up?" And most important, "Where do you eat?" When I told her that the hospital has a restaurant, she became very animated. "Daddy, this conversation has gone on too long!" Then she sprinted out of the room. "Eden! Eden! Do you know what?! They have a restaurant at the hospital!"

As she left, I realized that my bungled attempts to protect them had yet again proved foolhardy. Worse, I had failed to remember the one admonition we had most often flung their way: Use your words. Sure enough, as soon as we described where I had been going, their anxieties disappeared.

And I was reminded of one of my favorite messages from the Bible, from the opening of Genesis. Before there is order, there is chaos. Before there is light, there is darkness. And what is the only force strong enough to overcome that disorder? What does God use to create the world?

He uses words.

13

CHRONICLES OF THE LOST YEAR

volume IV

December 1

Dear Friends and Family,

Waves of wind, rain, and Arctic chill have passed through
Brooklyn in recent weeks and the leaves are finally off the
giant maple tree that shades our tiny backyard. With the
shortened days and vagaries of a brownstone's heating,
we now face the paradox of winter: the branches are bare
outside our windows but more light makes it into our
home.

One morning recently I found myself making a series of
lists. The first covered all the parts of my body that ached
or pained or had something wrong with them. I got so

overwhelmed I stopped counting at thirty. The second
list mentioned all the times I had cried in the previous
few weeks. This tally included a few pieces of bummer
news, at least one occasion of self-pity, a bout of agony
at the pain I was causing my family, and a tearful bit of
anticipation at receiving a friend's news that she was
cancer-free after five years. The final list counted all the
places I would rather have been that day. This list was
rather long.

It was my birthday. I was in the hospital.

As feared, the last few months have been challenging.
I passed into the belly of the chemo colossus and
experienced many of its most ferocious side effects. First,
I got an ear infection, followed by pneumonia, and had to
forgo several weeks of treatment. Then, twice in the span
of three weeks I was hospitalized on five minutes' notice—
once for elevated Methotrexate toxicity in my kidneys; the
second when my white- and red-blood counts fell to near
zero, and I had no effective immune system.

My doctors considered these developments routine and
were not particularly alarmed, but they are evidence
that the regimen, as promised, is taking its cumulative
toll and making my body weaker. Also, the physical and
emotional challenges of spending four days in a hospital
cancer ward all twisted up in IV cords and pumped up

on steroids are considerable. At one point I wrote Linda: "It's so much worse than anyone will ever know."

Still, I managed to pass through this unpleasantness and am excited to be nearing the end of the four-plus months of preoperative chemotherapy. My doctors are giving me several weeks off to regain my strength before the surgery, which is scheduled for late December. At the moment, Dr. Healey is planning a fairly innovative, sci-fi procedure. He will cut out the eight or so inches of my left femur that houses the primary tumor, then replace it with a titanium prosthesis. He will also remove the parts of my thigh muscle that have been corroded by the cancer.

A plastic surgeon, Dr. Bebak Mehrara, will then remove most of my left fibula, which we're told is an extraneous bone that doesn't need replacing. He'll graft the fibula to the healthy parts of my left femur, then screw it to the prosthesis. He'll then reconnect the fibula's blood vessels to those in my upper leg. The idea is to take the inorganic object—the titanium—and fuse it with an organic object—the fibula—to make the resulting construct as strong as possible. To give you an idea of how rare this is: Dr. Healey told us he has only done this procedure twice. But for what it's worth: One was on the special teams coach of the Jets, and as those in the New York area know, Gang Green's special teams have done quite well this year!

Following the surgery, I'll face several weeks of intensive, in-patient recuperation before being thrust almost immediately back into postoperative chemo, which should last another three months. At that point, with my body likely depleted and my mobility impaired, I'll begin physical therapy. As I've been referring to all this since July, I'm looking at The Lost Year.

So how are you holding up? I'm wobbly, at best. A few times in recent weeks, as I passed through rocky moments, I've wondered whether there is some correlation between cellular weakness and emotional sensitivity. The feebler I get the more acutely I feel the pain, especially emotionally. When my mother-in-law called me one night in the hospital a few weeks back and told me she thought the girls were suffering in my absence, I put down the phone and bellowed into my hands. There's a reason a primal scream is called a primal scream. Some fears are primordial.

Still, for the most part, we continue to take the hits, adjust our sights, and alter our expectations. Linda, in particular, has felt squeezed at times by having a husband in a hospital room across the river and two three-year-olds at home. She canceled her trips abroad, held conference calls from her cell phone in the chemo clinic, and struggled with my sometimes stoic silence.

The issue of how much discomfort to share with her and others who are already overburdened by caring for me has been a puzzle. One night Linda lay down on our bed and announced I simply had to share more of my struggle with her. I told her I was only keeping quiet to protect her, but when she insisted, I unloaded my catalog of minor ailments and anxieties. She became so rattled she didn't sleep for two days. Stoicism does have its virtues.

But a few of the dates that meant the most to me this fall did occur during "up days" in my treatment. Foremost among these was Linda's annual fund-raising gala for Endeavor. The event, which raises money for Linda's pioneering work supporting high-impact entrepreneurs in emerging countries, is like having to plan a wedding that is plopped down in the middle of our lives every year: black tie, five hundred people, seating charts, sensitive egos, and high-stakes toasts.

To add to the pressure, I was hospitalized as late as seventy-two hours before the event. But at the last hour my bone marrow rallied, and, in one of the few benefits of having lost so much weight, I was able to tuck myself into my wedding tux at the weight for which it was originally tailored. I even ditched my crutches for the night and strutted through my responsibilities as Endeavor's First Man. As Linda radiantly spoke of her organization's amazing accomplishments this year, and as

Endeavor's chairman, Edgar Bronfman Jr., paid tribute
to her incredible hard work even during her personal
struggle, I was hardly the only person raining tears in the
room.

For all the joy of this event, some warning signs did
emerge for future years—and I'm not referring to fund-
raising. I'm referring to fashion. We have a category
of marital accessory in our household that if I felt I
had any standing at all as a relationship guru, I would
recommend for all successful marriages, and that is: The
Gala Dress, otherwise known as The Thing About Which
I Don't Ask—Where It Came From, What It Looks Like,
How Much It Cost.

I've been quite proud of my hands-off attitude over the
years, but this year I realized I might have to change my
policy. The girls were quite excited by all the effort put
into Mommy's appearance and managed to get their own
nails done, too, at the Dashing Diva up the street. They
were even jazzed to see Daddy in his "tup-xedo." But
as I was leaving for the event, they announced: "Next
year we're going to get Gala Dresses, too!" Uh-oh. The
Domino Theory is back—and this time it seems to be
working.

The big picture. As you can see, cancer is not linear. Our
lives rock unaccountably—and unpredictably—among

moments of hardship, stress, joy, pride, laughter, and exhaustion. There is profundity to explore, but also laundry to do. Someone asked me recently whether the "up days" of chemo, following the "down days," suddenly seem beautiful and full of hope. Maybe, but I'm usually too busy unclogging the sink.

In that regard, we are very grateful for the many hours, afternoons, and weekends that our families and friends have spent helping us endure, and enjoy, this time. A special thank-you to the Class of 1983 at the Savannah Country Day School for taking time out of our reunion to send such robust best wishes. And our warmest embrace to all those who have sent nourishment, diversion, cards, and prayers. We have composed thank-you notes many times over in our heads. Please bear with our bad manners and know that we feel your support.

After five months, I have (mostly) accepted that I cannot anticipate or design how I will feel on any given day. One of my mottoes has become: "No excuses. No apologies. No planning." If someone makes me a giant bowl of chicken soup with matzah balls and I have a sudden craving for marinated artichokes and Milk Duds, I go with my craving. If someone flies in from Kazakhstan and cancels a lunch date with Mayor Bloomberg to come for a visit and I need a nap, I take the nap. I only wish selfishness was more fun!

As we head into the holiday season, the one list we know that is longer than ever is the one that contains all the things for which we are thankful. And if we've learned anything during this process, it's to take a moment to share that list with those who are on it. Recently I was speaking to a friend who had lost her father before her first birthday. The one thing she most missed from her father, she told me, was letters directly from him. My friend's older sister had received some, but she had not, because she was only a baby. My friend shared with me that every year she takes time to write a letter directly to each of *her* children telling them how much she loves them.

I can think of no better holiday wish from us to you. So in this season of anxiety and hope, may your home be filled with health, your lists with joy, and your letters with love.

And please, take a walk for me.

Love,

Bruce

·14·

BEN

Tend Your Tadpoles

FOR AS LONG AS I can remember, I kept an inventory in my head. I never gave it a name. I never wrote it down. The list contained the names of people who would come to my side in the case of an emergency, no matter the circumstances, no questions asked. If I got into trouble, I would just call one of these people and he (or she) would hop on a plane, or bail me out, or write the check, or hold my hand. And every time I made the list one name was at its top.

He was the friend who was always there, back before the memories begin. He was the friend who lived around the corner, who sat next to me at lunch, who assured me that some girl really did like me. He was the friend who traded his (forbidden) Rice Krispies treat for my (boring) Milano cookie, who helped make that epic Hot Wheels track that looped, Evel Knievel–like, down the stairs, around his mother's antique breakfront, and over the toilet. The thing really could have been in *The Guinness Book of World Records* if the dog hadn't knocked it over.

He was the friend whose birthday I never forget and whose childhood phone number I still remember. Who always looks eight to me, no matter the pounds, the gray hair, or the teenagers of his own.

He's the friend I have nothing in common with except that we grew up together.

Yet sure enough, when I got sick, he was the friend I had to call. And in that way you're always connected to that friend, even when you can't explain it; he was the friend that on the weekend when I was at my lowest—my birthday in the hospital—he was also at his bottom. His high school sweetheart, his wife of twenty years, the mother of his two children, sat him down and announced, "I'm leaving you."

He was the friend who then didn't tell me for six months because he didn't want to worry me.

———

THIS IS WHAT BEN Edwards wrote in my second-grade yearbook:

Bruce, Have a happy safe summer! I might come down to the beach to see you!!!!! You are very nice and kind. Love, Ben

The next year he added my nickname but cut out the love.

Tweddy Bear, I like you! Ben

The year after that he was downright cool.

Have a nice time at the beach. Ben

Not a single exclamation mark!

His school photos during those years show far less change. He always had the freckled cheeks, the innocent eyes, and the thin, straight hair with a gaping cowlick over his forehead. With his boy-next-door shirts and all-American style he could have stepped from the pages of a comic book. He was the Archie of our class.

Ben's small-town values were hard earned. His father, an obstetrician and gynecologist, was raised in Claxton, Georgia, home of the infamous boxed fruitcake more loved in truck stops than in restaurants. Its population in the year we were born was 2,672. Ben's mother was from nearby Brooklet, whose population was one-fifth that. I asked Ben whether his father had ever adapted to city life after moving to Savannah.

"I think Dad is still more of a country person," he said. "His favorite pastime is working in the yard. He's not into city-ish things like Starbucks, museums, and dining spots. He'd just as soon have fried chicken at the deli. He doesn't drink. He always goes to church. Heck, he wanted to own a gas station until Granny made him go to med school."

Dr. Edwards was deeply loving as a father. "To this day," Ben said, "he puts his arm around me. I put my arm around him, and we lie in bed watching TV."

But he could also be strict.

"I remember once when Joe was sixteen," Ben said, referring to his older brother. "We were in the den, Dad came home one Friday night and asked Joe to take out the trash. Joe said, 'Okay, I'll get it.' Twenty minutes later, Dad came back and asked him again. 'Dad, I told you I'll get it,' Joe said. Twenty minutes later, Dad came back again. 'Son, take out the trash now or I'm going to spank you.' Joe stood up and said, 'Dad, I'm bigger than you are. You're going to spank me?'

"Dad grabbed him by the shirt and said, 'Son, let me tell you one damn thing. You may be taller than me, but I will always have enough in my pocket to pay somebody to spank you, so I suggest you take the trash out.' Then he turned and walked away. Joe stood there for a second, then looked at me. 'I'm going to take the trash out.'"

Unlike his father, Ben was always attracted to city pleasures. Food, wine, nightlife, the annual Vegas weekend. He followed his father into medical school, then moved with his wife to Memphis and San Diego. But he couldn't resist the extended family and sweet-tea lifestyle of the South.

"I think there's a genuine goodness that runs through people here," he said. "I'm not saying people in the North don't have it. But you sit in a bar in California, and people are nice, but not genuinely nice. You sit in a bar in Georgia, and that person will end up going out with you that night, or giving you a ride somewhere, or inviting you over the next day for a barbecue."

"Why is that?" I asked.

"Things just move slower," he said. "You don't have as many people trying to . . . win."

"Unless it's football," I said.

"In which case you better win!" he said.

I told him that one of the most moving things about getting sick was how Savannah had rallied. Our classmates, parents, even onetime socialites who ignored me as a child, suddenly formed a scrum and tried to lift my entire family from afar.

"It's the Southern thing," Ben said. "Loyalty. Honesty. Friendship."

And these are the qualities I wanted Ben to impart to my girls. He would convey the importance of being from a place. How you carry that place with you wherever you go. How you keep coming back to it time and again no matter how long you live. "This is where your daddy came from," he would tell the girls. "This is where you come from, too."

Ben would teach them how to remember.

Our friendship started when we were five. "My earliest memory of you," Ben said, "is our holding hands, walking into kindergarten." He remembered our touch football games in the backyard and the time I defended him in fifth grade when he believed that Sharon Stubbs had a crush on him, but Charles Schwarz said she didn't and told Ben to be mean to her.

But his most vivid recollection was the most touching.

"In the fourth grade, we used to lay down on the carpet and read," he said. "One time, I was picking my nose and putting it into my mouth. Everybody was making fun of me, but you didn't break a sweat. You said, 'Ben, everybody is watching you pick your nose.' I looked up and everybody was pointing and laughing. The next two weeks, everyone made fun of me, but you didn't say a word."

"Thirty-five years later, this is what you remember!?"

"Your best friend was picking his nose and putting boogers in his mouth, and it didn't change anything with you. It comes back to loyalty."

I asked him why he thought we were friends.

"It starts off with proximity," he said. "Then, as we went along, we had similar interests, but we weren't into one-upmanship. You were obviously more artistic with plays and things like that, while I was always better than you in sports. But whatever you did, I did. And whatever I did, you did. Even if we didn't want to do it."

But for all our similarities, we had one gaping difference, and after race, it was the biggest one you could have in the South at that time.

Ben was Christian. I was Jewish.

In our talk, Ben alluded to it several times. My family ate different foods because we were Jewish. We lit candles and drank wine on Friday nights because we were Jewish.

Yet this difference was the source of our most powerful bonding experience: Every December I went to his house and helped decorate their Christmas tree. I loved the ritual of it, the colored lights and angels, the feeling of being included. When Ben's mother wrote me after I got cancer, she began with a beautiful thought: "When I see Ben, I think of you. You two were a great team." It ended with a question: "Do you remember helping us decorate our Christmas tree?"

Unlike some Jews, we didn't have a Christmas tree growing up; Linda and I don't have one today. But in a small way, my experience with the Edwardses' tinsel helped prepare me for the interfaith world I would later enter. Ben believes it shaped his life in even bigger ways.

"If you asked me what I think are my good traits," Ben said, "I would say first, hanging out with people who are different from me. I'm not saying I was perfect, or when I was in college I didn't chime in when people were making fun of others, just so I could be part of the crowd. But I have always been very accepting of diversity. It doesn't matter if you're black, white, Jewish, Christian, gay, lesbian, transvestite."

"Where did you learn that?"

He didn't pause. "The exposure to your family. I'm not giving you the whole credit, but I think you deserve a lot. Because your family was vastly different from mine. The principles were the same, but the underlying cultures were totally different. The Pop-Tarts versus the Milano cookies. The fun house versus the more serious, more artistic, more save-the-world house.

"You told me once I was your baseline American boy," he continued. "I went to college. I got a job. I married my high school sweetheart—" He caught himself. "And now I'm getting divorced. I guess I *am* fitting the pattern!

"But seriously," he continued. "Y'all aren't. None of your family is what I would consider Southern normalcy. But that diversity changed me and subtly became my baseline for what is American today."

Ben then shared a story I had never heard before. After high school, Ben went to the University of Georgia and joined a fraternity. In his sophomore year, he and his fraternity brothers were talking about rushes. "I was sitting with two guys I had known for a year, and someone made the comment, 'Oh, but he's Jewish. Do we really want a bunch of them in the fraternity?' And maybe I was naive, but I had never heard anybody say something derogatory like that. 'What are you *talking* about?' I said. 'Oh, you know, they're not like us,' the guy said. And I just ripped his head open. 'How do *you* know?' I said. 'Name me your Jewish friends.'

"We voted the guy into our fraternity."

———

BEN'S LOST YEAR BEGAN some months before mine, when his cousin Raul called him one day at work. Raul had grown up three doors down from me on Lee Boulevard, and his son, then thirteen, had an unusual growth in his leg. Ben, a bone radiologist, looked at the MRI. "Holy crap!" he thought. "This is an osteosarcoma. It's probably the only one in my entire life I will ever see."

"And what was the next beat in your mind?" I asked.

"He's going to die."

Over the next year, as "Little Raul" went through treatment and surgery, the community that later rallied around me rallied first around him. They catered meals. They decorated his house at Christmas. The entire seventh-grade class of boys shaved their heads in his honor.

Then, just as Little Raul was recovering, Ben got a similar call from me.

I asked him what he thought when he heard my diagnosis. He stammered for a second. "I thought the same thing," he said. "How does such badness happen to such good people. You get tired of it. When I biopsy patients, I can tell you whether it's going to be malignant just by how nice the person is. The nicer they are, the more malignant it's going to be. The pieces-of-dirt jerks could have the nastiest-looking lesion, and it will be an infection. A sweet little lady, she'll have pancreatic cancer. It's a running joke in the CAT scan department."

"And in that call, did you have the next beat?" I asked.

"Absolutely. I thought, 'Shit, my best friend's going to die.'"

"So it's twenty years from now," I said, "my daughters come to see you. They say, 'Nobody knew our daddy longer than you.' Where would you take them?"

"That's hard," Ben said, "because every place I can think of someone else would already have thought of." He mentioned Tybee Island and our school. "In the end, I think I would take them to that nasty creek behind your house where we used to catch tadpoles."

"The canal!" I said. "I haven't thought about that place in years."

The Hampstead Canal wasn't much of a canal at all; it was more of a drainage ditch filled with the lowest forms of life—algae, tadpoles, adolescent boys. It wasn't six feet wide, but to us it was the Amazon. One spring we started corralling tadpoles and trying to raise them into frogs. We put them in a plastic tub in our garage. They would sprout limbs and become vaguely frog-ish before stinking up the house so badly they had to be let loose.

"So what could Eden and Tybee possibly learn from the canal?" I asked.

"It's where we came from," he said. "It was a skanky and disgusting place. We never should have been there. Yet it's where we learned to be ourselves. It was home."

As he spoke I realized that Ben, that friend I barely knew, that friend I rarely saw, that friend who had prompted me to make that list of people I would call in an emergency only because I needed a way to name his role in my life, had hit on one of the deepest truths of all.

He was my tadpole.

He was that friend who was there at the beginning, who regardless of what had happened in between, returned at a moment of possible ending to remind me where we both started: two squiggly boys in a drainage ditch trying to cultivate arms and legs to hop off into the world.

And what I discovered in talking to Ben is what I learned time and again during my "Lost Year": As important as place is to my identity, I hadn't fully mined the roots of my geography; as vital as people are to my life, I hadn't truly plumbed the depths of my lineage. I hadn't read my grandfather's memoirs, delved into my father's past, or quizzed my friends about the headwaters of their lives. I had been content with the half-known and the unsaid.

I had avoided the canal.

And only by plunging into my past did I discover all

the nourishment that was floating in the water. As my girls liked to sing when they crossed the low bridge to Tybee Island, "And you'll always know your neighbor / And you'll always know your pal / If you've ever navigated on the Erie Canal."

Navigate the canal.

Tend your tadpoles.

You never know when you might need a pal.

15

BE A COLLECTOR

THE DIBNER LIBRARY OF THE History of Science and Technology is tucked in a remote corner of the ground floor of the Smithsonian's National Museum of American History in Washington, DC. I walk past a display of Julia Child's kitchen and an exhibition of illustrated Bibles, enter a small antechamber, lock my bag in a cubby, and go through a glass door.

Inside is a modest reading room, with six tables and lamps. On the wall hangs a portrait of Eli Whitney, the young Yale graduate who moved to Savannah in 1783 and invented the cotton gin. I am here to examine the collection of another Yale graduate with ties to Savannah.

The librarian carries out five volumes of loose-leaf eight-and-a-half-by-eleven-inch onionskin paper, hand-

typed in red and black ink, bound in black paperboard
binders. She places the first volume on a book stand. I
slip on a pair of white cotton gloves and open the cover.
Inside is a one-page bio of the author.

> Dr. Benjamin S. Abeshouse was born February
> 7th, 1901, in New Haven, Connecticut. He
> graduated from New Haven High School;
> attended Yale University, graduated 1921, then
> entered Yale Medical School graduating 1924.

The bio goes on to outline my grandfather's medical career, culminating in his rise to chief of urology at
Baltimore's Sinai Hospital in 1945. It mentions his three
children, along with 120 academic articles he wrote. It
ends with this statement: "He had various hobbies, i.e.,
collecting antiques, miniature ivories and statues; but his
pride, gathered in these volumes, was the world's largest
collection of epitaphs, 9,000 in total, which he and Mrs.
Abeshouse accumulated over a period of thirty years."

I was shaking. These pages were the closest I had
come to the man who died three years before I was born
and for whom I was named.

I was nervous. There was something ghostly about
learning during a year when my most pressing fear was
death that the figure who had hovered over my childhood had spent his entire adulthood collecting tombstone farewells.

And I was surprised. From the minute I turned the first page of these writings, any distance creepiness slipped away, and I was overwhelmed by a feeling of recognition, even kinship.

———

A PHOTOGRAPH DEFINED HIM while I was growing up. It hung outside my room and depicts him in profile, wearing a starched white tie and morning coat around a timpani chest. He seems poised for debate at Oxford. His face is round, even cherubic, with Harry Potter spectacles and thin hair, cleanly parted, waxed to his head. He hs a boy's innocence and a man's seriousness. Give him the floor, he would outargue you. Puncture him, and a flood of vulnerabilities would rush out.

I never noticed that vulnerability when I was a child. Instead, Bucky Abeshouse was so exalted he could have been a Roman emperor. His chiseled face belonged on an ancient coin—august, heralded, untouchable. I remember asking my father once about him; his reply seemed to cut off any questions: "He was a great man."

The truth, of course, was more complicated.

Bucky Abeshouse, too, grew up without a dad. He was the youngest of nine children from parents who emigrated from Vilna, Lithuania. His father, Abraham, died when he was two months old, leaving his mother to raise her kids while running a corner grocery. Bucky was the first in his family to attend college, and went to Yale at a time when Jews were not allowed to live on campus. After medical school, he relocated to Baltimore to train with a well-known urologist.

Urology in the 1920s was a young profession, and Bucky rose quickly. He penned academic articles on everything from urinary tract sarcomas to testicle surgery to "inflammation of the bladder due to the presence of a foreign object (a pencil)." He pioneered research into renal dyes and kidney dialysis.

And he was always writing. He wrote a book of popular history discussing the genital and urinary diseases of famous men, from Isaac Newton to Woodrow Wilson. Called *Troubled Waters* (a pun only a urologist could love), the book includes chapters on Ben Franklin's bladder stones and Napoleon's urinary tract infections.

My grandfather's expertise in male reproduction led to his having a comfort with sexuality that seems, at a minimum, uncommon for his era. He collected replicas of the *Manneken Pis*, the famed Belgian bronze sculpture of a naked boy urinating into a fountain. Bucky even molded a similar sculpture himself and recruited my ten-year-old mother to pose with a garden hose between her legs. In one reproduction that a friend lugged home from Europe, the boy's penis was fully erect. My grandmother, Carrie, placed it over the kitchen sink, using the boy's engorged phallus to store her wedding ring while she washed the dishes.

And in a fascinating career move that my mother didn't know about for more than seventy years, my white-tie-wearing grandfather wrote the introduction to a popular sex guide that was published in 1936. *The Single, the Engaged, and the Married* was so successful it was still in print twenty years later. The book says that sexual relations should be more openly discussed and enjoyed, and does so by advocating the notion that as one advances from single to engaged to married, a greater amount of sex will result. Maybe for you, Grandpa!

My mother was born the year the book was published, which raises the tantalizing possibility that Bucky was writing his essay at the time she was conceived. His piece may be the closest thing to a *Back to the Future* moment of witnessing my own origins I'll ever have. It suggests that in the middle of the Great Depression, my otherwise formal grandparents were, as the rappers like to say, knockin' da boots.

———

THE WORLD'S LARGEST COLLECTION of epitaphs is divided into five, carefully subdivided volumes. Book I contains the inscriptions of famous figures—pharaohs, poets, philosophers, kings. Book II gathers epitaphs based on cause of death—poisonings, railroad accidents, bee stings, burns, electrocutions, falling anchors, diarrhea, hangings. There's an entire chapter on unusual deaths. "The manner of her death was thus / She was druv over by a bus." There's another on food. "This disease you ne'er heard tell on, / I died of eating too much melon."

Subsequent volumes gather epitaphs of centenarians, movie stars, and drunks. His list by professions is prodigious: clockmaker, coal heaver, collier, stagecoach driver, cricketer, coroner, cremationist. And that's just the *c*'s! He finds dozens of epitaphs for prostitutes. "Here lies the body of young Miss Charlotte, / Born a virgin, dies a harlot. / For sixteen years she maintained her virginity / And that's a record for this vicinity." He even uncovers advertisements for widows.

Sacred to the Memory of Jared Bates
Who died August the 6th, 1800
His widow, aged 24, lives at 7 Elm Street,
Has every qualification for a good wife,
And yearns to be comforted.

His final epitaph purports to be the inscription of Jesus. "Therefore being satisfied with his life and faith, give him eternal happiness through grace."

It took me six hours to turn every one of the collection's 1,500 pages. I may be the only person other than Bucky (and Carrie, who typed them) who ever did.

My first impression was that the collection, while clearly a life's passion, may also have been an obsession. Bucky Abeshouse had a great mind, an astonishing knowledge of history, and a wicked sense of humor that I wish I had heard. And boy did he have follow-through! Robert Ripley of *Believe It or Not!* fame accumulated 5,000 epitaphs by the time of his death; Bucky Abeshouse had 9,000. His work is meticulous, but also encyclopedic, in both the best and worst senses of the word. There's very little perspective. No effort to explain his methodology. No attempt to make sense of what he gathered. There's no forest. Only trees.

With no overview, the only clue to Bucky's motivation is a one-and-a-half-page manifesto that appears at the start of Book 1. Labeled "Preface on Hobbies by Dr. Benjamin S. Abeshouse," it says the public should find it inspiring and consoling that physicians seek creative outlets for their noteworthy talents beyond their profession. "These artistic manifestations should be considered as safety valves," he writes, "offering an outlet to the nervous tension of those constantly walking in the footsteps of death. A romantic expression may be just the thing to remove the embitterment."

His conclusion is that others should follow the same path. "Be a collector, make a garden, have a hobby."

My mother used virtually the same words when we were kids. We might call it the Abeshouse Absolute.

AFTER LEAVING WASHINGTON, I drove to Arlington Cemetery in Baltimore to visit my grandfather's grave site. A beautiful stretch of grass contains row after row of unadorned graves. In the middle, an arched gray headstone is chiseled with the name ABESHOUSE. A small footstone bears his name, along with the boiler-plate BELOVED HUSBAND & FATHER. In the middle is the winged staff of Hermes, the symbol of medicine.

There is no epitaph.

After three decades of gathering every imaginable inspiration, Bucky Abeshouse chose none as his legacy. Maybe he couldn't decide. Maybe he died so suddenly he didn't have time. Or maybe, as my brother put it, he had writer's block.

Either way, as I stood there, I began reflecting on the parallel lives of Bucky Abeshouse and my paternal grandfather, Edwin Feiler Sr. In many ways, they could not have been more different. One was from the urban North; the other the rural South. One was a scholar and collected epitaphs in Latin; the other played blackjack, trapped squirrels, and fished. One was a teetotaler; the other drank moonshine.

But in crucial ways, they had deep similarities. Both were the first in their families to attend college, and each went on to earn professional degrees, in effect isolating them from their closest relatives. Both initiated decades-long literary projects that few would ever see (or hear). Both abstained from joining the types of civic and community institutions that would later define their children—arts groups, political parties, volunteer organizations.

Both were self-made men. And both, in a crucial sense, were alone.

I felt an allegiance with the loneliness of Bucky

Abeshouse, a lion whose mane was always draped around my shoulders. As a writer, I felt the kinship of the solitary pursuit. With an output of four academic articles a year, a book of popular history, and his collection of epitaphs, Bucky Abeshouse sacrificed himself to the calling of words. My mother remembers him sitting in the den every night, surrounded by three radios and a television set, all tuned to different sporting events. "You could walk in at any time," she said, "and he could tell you the score for every game."

I must say, it sounds familiar. He would have felt right at home in my office, with three news sites open on my computer, stacks of books on my desk, and ESPN on the flat-screen TV.

Even deeper, Bucky was clearly drawn to epitaphs because his profession exposed him to mortality. He described this feeling in his opening essay as "walking in the footsteps of death." But he also must have felt the lure because of the loss of his own father. Perhaps spending so much time in the company of ghosts drew him closer to his dad.

His searching certainly drew him closer to me, especially when I also felt the pull of death—and the loneliness that comes with it. Perhaps the most disturbing aspect of getting sick as a young person is the profound isolation that comes from thinking about dying when so few people around you are doing so.

Standing at his grave, in my own year of epitaphs, I

felt for the first time that Bucky Abeshouse wasn't just an untouchable portrait on the wall. He was real. In our shared passion for language and our joint interest in mortality, I had finally found in myself the part of him that was there all along.

And I was reminded of the common message that both my grandfathers seemed to be sending: Don't disappear, don't withdraw. Turn away from the briefs, the records, and the pages and turn toward the people who are just out of view.

16

CHRONICLES OF THE LOST YEAR

volume V

February 3

Dear Friends and Family,

Relentless torments of snow and ice have battered
Brooklyn in recent weeks, leaving the streets and
sidewalks a chalky, salty mess, and our creative ways of
keeping kids occupied while indoors tapped out long
ago. But even as winter slogs toward its halfway mark,
if you look outside in the late afternoons, you can begin
to detect that the light lasts a little longer, hinting that
relief is on the way.

There are very few days in one's life that you know, in
advance, are going to be momentous. December 23

was one of those days for me. I awoke before dawn and arrived at the hospital at 5:45 A.M. for the beginning of what would be a fifteen-hour surgery to salvage my left leg. An orthopedic fellow arrived to sign my thigh, and at 7:30 A.M. I was wheeled down the longest hallway I had ever seen. (I later determined that the world's longest hallways are probably all outside surgery rooms, and I learned that this hallway, long even by hospital standards, has been nicknamed "The Green Mile.")

Inside, the OR was a mix of high-tech television screens; a swarm of nurses and attendants; a man with a large, astronautlike glass bubble around his head; and a twelve-foot-long table overflowing with knives, scalpels, and prongs. There was enough equipment to cook a state dinner, though in this case the only thing being carved was me. In the last minutes before the anesthesia kicked in, my surgeon, Dr. John Healey, appeared over my table to tell me that the latest scans of my leg suggested that the tumor had been wiped out by the chemotherapy. "It's dead," he said. As he later told my family, "I wanted Bruce to go to sleep with a smile."

As I drifted into sleep Dr. Healey went to work, while Linda, my mom, and my brother waited anxiously outside. At 12:15 P.M. a nurse let them know that Dr. Healey was still resecting the cancerous material from my femur and thigh. At 2:50 P.M. they got a similar report,

and at 4:50 P.M. another. At 6:10 P.M., Linda, Andrew,
and my mother were escorted into a room where Dr.
Healey joined them five minutes later. "He's doing fine,"
Dr. Healey said. "I'm fine. That says it all."

In his patient, arresting manner, Dr. Healey spent the
next forty-five minutes outlining what he had done. First
he removed twenty-two centimeters of my left femur
(just shy of nine inches), as well as about a third of my
quadricep. The amount of muscle resected was less than
he had anticipated, and he was especially pleased that he
was able to save a key artery he had expected to have to
remove. "Bruce is going to love this," Dr. Healey said.
"The artery is called the profunda."

Dr. Healey then installed the specially crafted titanium
prosthesis into the gap in my femur, attached the
device to the remaining bone, and screwed the entire
contraption into place. Though we had expected this
prosthesis to mimic the shape of the femur, it's actually
a series of tubes, cubes, rods, and rings that appears
more akin to a shock absorber, though without the ability
to expand and contract. (My brother thinks it looks
more like the handle of a light saber from *Star Wars*.) Dr.
Healey was encouraged that the prosthesis fit snugly
into the good parts of my femur and likened the gap to
that between a boat and a dock: the closer one is to the
other, the easier it is for the healthy bone to make the

leap and grow into the prosthesis. Overall, Dr. Healey said he felt emboldened by the positive developments and pushed himself to take even more chances and be even more courageous. Asked if there were any surprises, Dr. Healey said, "Bruce has a very big leg!"

Though Dr. Healey's work was mostly done, mine was not. While Dr. Healey was briefing my family, the plastic surgeon, Dr. Mehrara, went to work on my lower leg. Dr. Mehrara removed a little more than nine inches of my left fibula, grafted it to my remaining femur, then screwed the fibula into the prosthesis. In order to keep the fibula alive, Dr. Mehrara removed four blood vessels from my calf and relocated them to my thigh. When he told my family about all this at 11:30 P.M., he, too, was upbeat. "Good bone; good vessels; no problem," Dr. Mehrara said. Dr. Healey returned near midnight to provide an exclamation point to this magnum day. "Believe it or not, I'm ecstatic," he said. As promised, Dr. Healey was the last man standing; as foretold, he was the hero of this war.

And then: the recovery. I woke up the next morning in a fog of narcotics, tubes, drains, and incoherence. I had thirty-one inches of stitches up the side of my left leg and no clue what had happened. Even more confusing, during the time I was on the operating table the doctors had forcibly shut my eyes with what must have been duct tape, and I woke up with a scratched cornea. No one could explain why such a high-tech operation had been marred by this low-tech methodology. An eye doctor arrived that evening—Christmas Eve—to test my sight; he stuck a miniature eye chart about six inches in front of my face. In my state, the whole thing appeared to bounce up and down like a trampoline. "I think you need glasses," the doctor said and thrust a monocle in front of my eyes. "I don't need glasses," I said desperately, "I don't need this test." Then I promptly threw up on him. Unflustered, he declared my scratched cornea the worst he had ever seen and ordered me not to open my right eye for three days!

Within days my sight had improved, I weaned myself off the morphine drip, and began to take stock of my body. In effect, I had two different wounds. The first was the thigh, which was grossly swollen, had two drains to reduce the swelling, and seventy-five stitches that stretched more than a foot and a half from my hip to my knee. The second was the calf, which had its own drain, was wrapped in a splint to prevent movement, and had thirteen inches of dissolvable stitches. The ortho team was responsible for the upper wound; the plastics team for the lower; and each side strenuously avoided commenting, inspecting, or even looking at the other wound. But they did continuously blame the other team for keeping me in bed. For a time it seemed as if my leg had become the United States before the Civil War—with my thigh the North; my calf the Confederacy; and my knee was the Mason-Dixon Line. The frustrating standoff needed Lincoln to restore the Union.

On the seventh day, Dr. Healey (after protesting that he was not as tall as Lincoln) finally broke the stalemate and provided a surprising diagnosis. I had eased past the possible complications of surgery more hastily than they expected, and my leg was simply not ready yet to begin rehabilitation. "I'm afraid you recovered too quickly," he joked.

Finally, on Day Eleven, I was allowed to sit up for the first time. "Your leg will swell; it will fill with blood; and it will turn purple," Dr. Healey warned. "Your head will throb; you'll get dizzy; and you'll faint." He was right! Over the next twenty-four hours I slowly made it out of bed, into a wheelchair, and into my new life. On Saturday, January 3, twelve days after I arrived, I was finally sent home. It took an ambulance, a fire truck, two crews, a stretcher, and a near overdose of painkillers to get me out of Manhattan, into Brooklyn, up a flight of stairs, and into my bed. The girls came upstairs and swarmed around me. We had reached the end of phase two of our yearlong war.

And we did so on a high of positive news. The day before

releasing me, Dr. Healey had paid an unannounced visit to my hospital room. Linda and I were eating a mushroom and anchovy pizza she had smuggled onto the seventh floor. Dr. Healey had just come from the Tumor Review Board, he said, and had some news. The pathology showed that the chemo had been astonishingly successful, and the kill rate for my tumor was 100 percent. This result substantially increases the chances that the chemo killed the invisible cancers in my blood that have been our primary concern since July and likely improves my overall prospects. The normally reserved Dr. Healey could not contain his enthusiasm. "This is not a small skirmish," he said. "This is victory in a major battle." He then reached out and shook my hand.

Even with this burst of momentum, the following weeks proved extremely challenging. Back at home, the pain was intense, the inconvenience enormous, and the progress of regaining my strength and mobility far more tedious than I had feared. My days became consumed with drug regimens, bedpans, sponge baths, physical therapists, and my pitiful attempt at exercises designed to regain even nominal movement in my left leg. The simple act of turning over in bed would often leave me howling; going outside to visit the doctor required three people to assist me, including someone elevating my leg as I bumped down the stairs on my rear end like a toddler, out the door, and down the icy stoop. My orders call for no weight at all on my leg until Valentine's Day, followed by six weeks of 50 percent weight on my leg, then months of physical rehab to help me learn to walk again.

And to make our lives significantly more complex, ten days after being discharged from the hospital, I began three months of postoperative chemo. Suddenly I layered all the miseries of last fall—nausea, weight loss, low blood counts, and mental anguish—on top of the pain in my leg. I've been hospitalized once since that time and on more than one occasion found myself just crying out unexpectedly, "I don't want to have cancer anymore!"

But, of course, I don't have cancer anymore. We must live with the threat that it could return at any time, but for now, at least, I am cancer-free. The one strategic decision we made last summer was to delay the surgery for half a year in part to tell if my body would respond to the chemo. Boy did that decision pay off. The news from phase one was as good as we could have hoped; phase two, the surgery, also appears to have been a remarkable success. We are now well into phase three, and we do so with momentum and firmly focused on the future.

So how did everyone else bear up? Linda braved this unimaginable ordeal with more grace and good cheer than almost anyone else I can imagine. Our families rallied in extraordinary ways, kept the girls occupied, and spent all hours of the day and night, first at the hospital then at home, moving necessities to within arm's reach. My mother even sacrificed a few afternoons of vigil to beat me in *every single game* of gin rummy we played.

On one memorable afternoon five days after the surgery, we brought the girls to the hospital for a visit. I had worried about this occasion for months, eager not to traumatize them. I persuaded the nurses to unhook me from my IVs, ditched my gown for civilian clothes, covered up my wounds and all the scary equipment with sheets, and welcomed the girls into my bed. We had scripted the event down to the nanosecond. The girls gave me a gift, I gave them one, I read through *Curious George Goes to the Hospital,* then we whisked them away before they could take in too much information. Tybee was especially excited to meet Dr. Healey near the elevator, and when everyone got outside, Eden announced, "Thank you for taking us to the hospital, Mommy." Upstairs, I wept like a baby and proud father all at the same time.

With the passage of time, our lives have once more settled into a routine. With such a long lag since my pre-Thanksgiving chemo, my eyebrows and eyelashes returned in force, along with my military buzz cut, and the unwelcome addition of my first-ever five-o'clock shadow. The girls excitedly tracked my leg's evolution from stitches to scar and have come to relish their late-afternoon ballet performances in our bedroom. (The one mandatory note: tossing pretend flowers for the "grand finale" and pretend candy for the "encore.") Our little family once more is a unit—hobbled but moving forward.

We fully expect February and March to be challenging months. Linda is headed first to California, then later to India; I am surely heading back into the hospital. But I have promised the girls I will begin to walk about more freely by their birthday in mid-April and that my hair will grow back by this summer. On some days, these landmarks even seem close.

Until then, we take comfort that so many of you are taking this journey alongside us and know that even in the face of your own setbacks, standoffs, snowstorms, and heartaches, you'll take an afternoon with someone you love, think of the many blessings you've sent our way, and use our struggles to help you persevere a little more easily through this season of challenges.

And, of course, please take a walk for me.

Love,

Bruce

17

BEN THE SECOND

Live the Questions

BEN SHERWOOD WAS PUSHING ME in a wheelchair around the seventh floor of Memorial Sloan-Kettering hospital, looking for a place to talk. A month after surgery and back under twenty-four-hour care for a depleted immune system, I was haggard, immobile, and scared. I was in the one place I least wanted to be.

And Ben was where he had been from the beginning.

He was present.

From the moment of my diagnosis, Ben had peppered me with e-mails—two, four, ten times a day. He called from traffic jams, television studios, backyards playing catch with his son, treadmills where he was trying to lose weight through diet, exercise, and competition with me, even though I had an unfair advantage, since I was losing mine through chemotherapy. He flew from his home in Los Angeles to be at the hospital at 5:30 A.M. on the morning of my biopsy.

He was, as he liked to say, a soldier in my army.

We found an abandoned conference room. Ben rolled me to the head of the table and pulled up a chair. Though Ben was one of the first dads on my list, he was about to become one of the last to know. The reason: Ben is the friend who questions. He challenges assumptions and picks apart flaws. If some friends are cheerleaders, bulwarks, and backstops, Ben is the inquisitor. He's the drill sergeant making sure every decision is thought through and every emotion pure. *Push it! Push it! Just one more round. No pain, no gain!*

I had to be prepared.

I exhaled and read my letter.

Will you tell them what I would be thinking? Will you be my voice?

Ben choked up as I was reading. Tears streamed down his face. He was caught unprepared. "Oh, Brucie," he said.

Then he caught himself. "But I completely reject the premise," he said. "And I hereby tender my resignation."

It was a classic Sherwoodian thrust: Bold. In-your-face. Attacking the foundation.

But I knew it was coming and quickly parried. "But Linda wants you in my Council," I said.

He knew he could no longer resist. "In that case," he said, "I know the perfect place to take you."

———

ONE SURPRISING OUTCOME OF creating the Council of Dads was I unintentionally gave six men carte blanche to voice their opinions. Not so much about child rearing— my experience is that men are generally less judgmental about that (or at least less vocal with their judgments)— but about the Council itself. *The Council has to meet. The Council should never meet. We should take the girls somewhere. We should leave them alone for now.*

We should go fishing!

I hadn't really thought through these issues, and I was reluctant to prescript a set of rules. I was more interested in creating a well-balanced cabinet and letting life take its course.

But I quickly realized that part of the Council's magic was it put six men together and let them be, well, men. Their purpose was to help fill the Dad Space in the girls' lives. And for all the heavy breathing about my generation's equal parenting—Jeff's cuddling; Max's 2:00 A.M. diaper changes; David's biscuits—most people still think a father should perform certain functions. These have to do with boundary drawing and expectations setting, prodding and enforcing, listening and embracing. Whatever else they do, Dads these days are still expected to push, to shape, to voice a code of responsibility.

And in my Council, no one pushes harder, shapes more thoughtfully, or has a stronger voice than Ben Sherwood.

Ben is big. He has a big family—the larger-than-life grandfather, the towering father, the path-breaking older sister. He has a big résumé—the high school debating trophies, the Rhodes Scholarship, the multiple Emmys. He has a big body—the "unusually large, and misshapen head," as he puts it, the Kennedy cleft chin, the six-foot-four frame. If I were *his* height, I'd be in the NBA.

And he has a big heart.

On a gloomy morning in Los Angeles, he invited me to the backyard of his childhood home off Sunset Boulevard, to sit underneath the family's sycamore tree with white camouflage bark and broad, pea green leaves. "This tree is where my father and mother courted," he said, "where my sister and husband were married, where Karen and I were married, and where we gathered fifteen years ago to have a memorial service for my dad. My sister and I played here. My son plays here now. It's home base."

Place looms large in the Sherwood family tree. The flats of Beverly Hills were to him as the dunes of Tybee Island were to me.

"My grandfather, Ben the First, was a jeweler," Ben explained. "He wasn't educated, but he was a dynamic, charismatic, life-of-the-party figure who tormented family members with practical jokes, needled people, and pushed their buttons. I certainly inherited some of that."

His father, Dick, was quite different, a soft-spoken, studious man who would have preferred to be a professor or foreign service officer but whose father demanded that he pursue a professional degree. He became a litigator and eventually argued before the Supreme Court. But in a manner resonant with my own dad, Ben's father directed his deeper passions into what was known at the time as "building the institutions of the city." He was a classic, late-twentieth-century Wise Man.

"My father was a gentleman and a gentle man," Ben said. "But he was not his father. He was distant, uncomfortable with the direct expression of emotion. He was stoic. I remember being shocked the first time I saw him cry. I came into his bedroom after his mother died, and he immediately tried to compose himself."

He was also focused on family. "Dad's parenting style was to be present as much as possible, given the demands of his life. That meant he was here for breakfast and dinner, during which time it was expected that we would have a serious conversation about the world. My dad had a voracious curiosity. He ran a famous clipping service in which he dispatched yellow envelopes from his law firm with articles on some obscure topic from some esoteric publication, pertinent to someone's work or family. We all got them. In college I had stacks of unopened envelopes because I just couldn't keep up!"

At times Dick Sherwood's bookishness collided with his parenting, as when he played baseball with his son, using a mitt that had never been broken in and clumsily tossing the ball into the bushes. "Image: Dad, at the Roxbury Park Little League, in a sport coat and tie, reading the *New York Times* in the bleachers. When it was my turn to bat, the paper would come down. When I was done batting, the paper would come up."

Above all, Dick Sherwood led by gentle inquisition. "Dad's part was constantly testing our hypotheses. He would question every decision. He would make sure our ideas had been stress tested in the modern sense of 'Do you have answers that stand up to rigorous thought?' "

He even turned his passion into sport. "We often played a game called Box," Ben said. "He would ask a question, and at the end would be a box." Ben made a rectangle with his fingers to represent the ideogram. "He would say, 'In the United States, we have a president. In England, they have a . . . BOX.' He had this wonderful deep voice, so it came out BAAAWWWXX. And you had to fill in the box.

"My friends in college loved it when he showed up and boxed them," Ben said. "They would say, 'My topic is Mexican trade policy,' and he would say, 'The first president of Mexico to initiate trade with California was . . . BOX.' And my friends would be stumped! Barry Edelstein is the only person who ever reverse-boxed my dad, and my father couldn't fill it in. It was one of those amazing moments. 'Oh, my God, you've just knocked down the champ!' " (The question: "The original Sweeney Todd on Broadway was played by . . . BOX?")

"So what's the meaning of the game?" I asked.

"It's a way of thinking about things. A way of knowing things. A way of learning to ask questions about the world."

The game worked. Ben became a broadcast journalist, rising meteorically through prime-time news, nightly news, then morning news. In 1993, while working in Washington, Ben got a call one Friday evening from his mom. "Something has happened to Dad," she said. Dick Sherwood had been standing, reading the *Financial Times* at his secretary's desk, when he collapsed. He got up briefly, then collapsed again, at which point he was rushed to Good Samaritan Hospital in downtown Los Angeles, where doctors determined he had suffered a massive brain hemorrhage. He was sixty-four years old.

When Ben arrived the following day, his father was in a coma. "The doctor said to me, 'You need to hope that your dad does not recover from this, because if he wakes up, he will not be who he was.' And I remembered having a conversation with my dad, six months earlier, in which we talked about the brain, and he said that what gave him an advantage in the courtroom was that, in basketball terms, he was a half step ahead of everybody else. And that half step, that tiny increment, was what gave him the greatest joy in life.

"So I realized," Ben said, "that the next five days were not about his recovery. They were more about the family coming to terms with the fact that we would eventually have to unplug the machines, which we did."

"Did you say good-bye?"

"Yes. I was with my sister. I stroked his face. Kissed him good-bye. Said we would take care of Mom." He paused. "One of the peculiar things is that he was very much there. His heart was pounding. He had a beard from a week of not shaving. But, of course, he wasn't there."

"What do you most miss?"

"I don't miss the questions," Ben said. "He taught me how to ask those." His voice grew strained and thin, as if each level deeper of emotion sounded an octave higher.

"I miss his voice." He inhaled deeply. "I can still hear it." Ben was sobbing now, like a boy. Watching a man of such measure reduced to such essence offered a glimpse into the private conversation the two of them had shared over the arc of the question marks.

"He had a wonderful voice," Ben said. "The timbre. Which is why your project struck home with me, Brucie. Because if you weren't here, I would want your girls to be able to hear you and your voice. And not in the saddest moments. That's not when I miss my dad the most. In the happiest moments. The times of greatest joy are the times that are bittersweet because my dad's not here to enjoy them. To witness them. And to add his voice."

WHEN I MOVED TO New York in 1997 I started a weekly happy hour with two friends. We weren't joiners, so in a bid to save face we called it the No Name Happy Hour. It became a place for writers, editors, and television types to beat the city. About a year in, a friend announced, "I'm going to bring somebody new next week. You're going to either love him or hate him. His name is Ben Sherwood."

Ben in those days cut a particular swath through New York. He was tall. He was successful. He was single. He was stiff. He worked for NBC News all day; he wrote romantic novels all night. The onetime champion debater seemed uncomfortable in social situations unless there was a prescribed set of rules—the eight-minute constructive speech, the three-minute cross-examination, the four-minute rebuttal. He would have been ripe for a send-up on *Sex and the City,* and, considering he went on a few dates with a writer for the show, he might have been.

His first impression of me was skeptical. "I thought you were an intense talker, with a big personality, big hands, and big stories. I believed you were always on output, so it took me a while to realize how intensely sensitive you are to all the feedback around you. To recognize that you're also on input. I doubt we would have become the friends we are today if we both didn't listen intently."

Ben and I quickly formed a sort of round-the-clock running commentary about politics, girls, media, the Page Six creatures we wanted to puncture, the men we wanted to become. The only thing missing was sports. He sadly inherited his dad's disinterest in athletics.

Above all, we created one of the hardest things to create: a close male friendship later in life. And as he courted, married, and became a father, I watched the once starchy caricature morph into a warmer, fuller man.

What never changed during those years was his heart, or his mind.

He never stopped asking questions.

And it's that voracious, sometimes relentless, curiosity I wanted him to pass on to the girls. The commitment to unveiling the truth behind the spin. The thirst to acquire information, then rearrange it into something surprising and fresh. "If something happened in the news," Linda said, "and I wanted the girls to have an unexpected view of it as you would have given, I would send them to Ben."

Ben would teach them how to think.

Which is why it was no surprise, sitting under the tree, when I asked him what message he would share with my daughters if I were no longer alive, he pulled out his BlackBerry.

"I would share with them this quotation from Rainer Maria Rilke," he said.

Have patience with everything unresolved in
your heart. Try to love the questions themselves.
Do not seek the answers now, because you
would not be able to live them. And the point is
to live everything. Live the questions.

"It connects to BOX," Ben said. "It connects to my way of seeing things. It connects to who you are as a traveler. There's an African proverb that the man who asks questions is never lost. And I think that's very much your approach to walking the world, which is that you can be in the absolute most foreign place, most exotic place, most unrecognizable place, and if you ask questions you'll always be able to find your way. Confidence comes from the questions. So I would tell the girls to live their questions. Throw themselves passionately into the quest for new perspectives, just like their father, who would go anywhere in search of answers to his questions."

The sun had begun to burn off the morning gloom by now. A crow alighted on the tree. Ben's voice was no longer cracking. It was pure.

"What I love about the Council of Dads," he said, "is that if your girls are too young to hear your voice, you can surround them with voices that will, in the totality of symphony, create sounds of their father. No specific instrument does it. Sherwood's drum may be beating too loudly, or maybe Black's or Stier's will screw things up. But Linda will conduct the orchestra in such a way that the girls will hear enough music for you to be always present."

"So in that symphony of voices, what would you like your voice to be?"

"I think I would like to be the contrarian," Ben said. "The dissonant voice. I would like to be the note—not the false note, but the true note—that does not feel as if it fits into the music but is critical to making the piece perfect. Because that's the role we play in each other's lives. Which is, 'Everybody else says this. But what's Bruce going to say?' I've tested an idea. I've tested it. I think I've made it work. But he's going to ask a question that will make me go forward with greater confidence or take all the data and reprocess it in a completely different way.

"That gift is what I would like to share with Tybee and Eden," Ben said. "Because the people who live the answers have a lot more safety, a lot more security, and a lot more stability."

"And the people who live the questions are . . . BOX."

"Discoverers."

18

THE LAST FEW STEPS

Bonaventure Cemetery, just east of Savannah, has two side-by-side stone gates at its entrance. The gate on the left has two chiseled stone pillars capped with female figures cradling crosses. It is known as the Christian gate. The gate on the right has similar stone pillars topped with Stars of David. It's called the Jewish gate.

On a swampy, mosquito-plagued afternoon I drove through the Jewish gate, grabbed my crutches, and climbed the few steps to the visitors' center. Inside are sample stone carvings, assorted porcelain urns for ashes, and portraits of famous people buried here, including governors, ambassadors, and Confederate generals, along with Pulitzer Prize–winning poet Conrad Aiken and four-time Oscar-winning songwriter Johnny Mercer.

A sign tells visitors that Bonaventure's most famous resident, "The Bird Girl," a four-foot-two-inch bronze statue of a girl holding a bowl in each hand, has been relocated to a museum downtown. This little-known statue from an unheralded plot was featured on the cover of John Berendt's *Midnight in the Garden of Good and Evil.* The book's meteoric success inspired countless pilgrims to trek to Savannah, many of whom came to Bonaventure and began chipping off chunks of the statue's pedestal.

I gave the attendant my surname. She disappeared into a musty back room, then returned momentarily with six worn, yellowed cards. Each contained the name of someone interred at the cemetery, the date and place of the person's death, along with the date, style, and location of burial. The names were my great-grandparents, Daisy and Melvin Feiler; my great-great uncle Edwin Cohen; my grandparents, Aleen and Edwin Feiler; and my uncle Stanley Feiler.

I was amazed by how much information these cards revealed. My great-grandfather managed to be buried on the same day he died, July 18, 1952. My great-grandmother, who died on September 27, 1960, was relocated from Starkville, Mississippi, in time to be buried two days later. My uncle, whose body was donated to science, was buried seven months after his death, in April 2001. My uncle was cremated; my grandmother buried in a casket; my great-grandmother interred in a monarch vault. "It's a concrete container," the attendant explained. "Jews aren't usually buried in vaults, just dry ground. But things are always changing."

I thanked her, returned the cards, and stood up to leave.

"Are you going to visit your family?" she asked.

"Sort of," I said. "Really I came to visit my own grave site."

———

BONAVENTURE, OR "LOVELY PLACE," is one of the most storied settings in an otherwise storied city. Established as a rice plantation before the American Revolution, the wooded bluff above the Wilmington River became a private cemetery in 1846. The seller, U.S. Navy Commodore Josiah Tattnall, is said to have introduced the line "blood is thicker than water" into American history after aiding the British against the Chinese in 1859.

The cemetery's most distinctive feature is what *Harper's Magazine* in 1860 called it's "mournful avenue of live oak," a promenade of soaring evergreens called the king's trees because their hearty wood was once reserved for the Royal Navy. John Muir, the founder of the Sierra Club, who camped in Bonaventure for five days in 1867, called the specimens "the most magnificent planted trees I have ever seen. The main branches reach out horizontally until they come together over the driveway, while each branch is adorned like a garden with ferns, flowers, grasses, and dwarf palmettos."

Nearly every branch of these grand oaks is draped in silvery, beardlike skeins of *Tillandsia,* or Spanish moss, which shrouds the entire grounds with a funereal air. A cousin of the pineapple, the exotic garlands swing and sway with every motion of the wind, wrote a visitor in 1859, "not unlike the effect produced by the tattered banners hung from the roofs of Gothic cathedrals as trophies of war in olden time."

Covering over 160 acres, Bonaventure was part of the rural cemetery movement of the nineteenth century in which burial grounds were relocated from crowded church backyards to plush, garden-style paradises, where the deceased would retire close to nature and the grieving would be uplifted by the blooms. These "cities of the dead" were designed to be places of hope, not sadness, where death was no longer macabre but a state of "silent slumber," "sweet repose," or "eternal sleep."

Forerunners of modern-day parks, cemeteries became desired leisure destinations where people brought carriages, picnics, and amorous intention. Anyone who courted in Bonaventure on a Sunday, it was said, was sure to marry. Bonaventure is so lovely, wrote one observer, that "Death is robbed of half its horrors."

I searched out three family plots before heading to my own. The first belonged to Johnny Mercer, whose mournful ballad "Moon River" is Savannah's unofficial anthem. The lyricist of more than 1,500 songs, and cofounder of Capitol Records, is buried alongside his wife, Ginger, and other family members. The stones bear his song titles: "My Mama Don Tol' Me" for his mother; "You Must Have Been a Beautiful Baby" for his wife; "And the Angels Sing" for himself.

Conrad Aiken is also buried alongside his parents, though the overtones are less pleasant. When Aiken was eleven, he awoke one morning to hear his parents arguing. His father then shot his mother and turned the pistol on himself. The future poet laureate of the United States ran barefoot across the street to the police station. "Papa has just shot Mama and then shot himself."

The elder Aikens' graves are marked with a single monument, while the troubled writer, who went on to edit the Harvard literary magazine with T. S. Eliot and lived around the world before returning to Savannah, is buried under a granite bench to encourage visitors to stop and enjoy a drink. The bench contains an inscription that my brother has adopted as his Internet alias. One day Aiken saw a ship named *Cosmos Mariner* sailing into Savannah. Enchanted, he checked the paper for its routing, only to find a boilerplate entry saying no information was available. The entry became his epitaph.

COSMOS MARINER

DESTINATION UNKNOWN

The third grave I visited was more personal to me.

Jack Leigh was the photographer who took the image of the "Bird Girl" that appeared on the cover of *Midnight in the Garden of Good and Evil*. A native Savannahian and a graduate of my high school, Jack dreamed of being a painter but abandoned that for photography. After apprenticing widely, he returned to Savannah, took a haunting shot of a swan in the city's most touristed fountain, and believed for the first time that he could see his hometown in a fresh way. That image now hangs on our bedroom wall in Brooklyn Heights, a symbol of a private stroll Linda and I took around the fountain moments after we were married.

Jack went on to publish five books of precisely focused, finely observed images of dying worlds along the rivers, swamps, and inland waterways of Georgia's low country. In 2003, in his early fifties, Jack was diagnosed with terminal colon cancer. He longed to spend his final weeks in the place he loved most, Tybee Island. My parents offered him their beach house. Jack experienced his waning days in the place where I spent my weaning ones. When I was struck early with cancer, the parallels with my longtime friend, who also had two daughters at home, were painful. I was curious about his state of mind as the end of his life neared.

"Jack's primary work as a documentary photographer," said Susan Patrice, his ex-wife, who spent the final months at his side, "was really the work of being an open human being who could show up in any situation and be truly open and engaged. And while you're developing that skill as an artist, you also develop it as a human.

"What I found remarkable," Susan continued, "is that as we were driving out to Tybee after Jack had been in the hospital for months, he kept saying, 'Slow down. I've forgotten how beautiful the world really is. Do you see it? Do you see it?' I kept thinking, 'He sees it because he's visited death, but also because he's cultivated this capacity to see. He may not be strong enough to lift the camera, but the camera has become irrelevant.'"

Jack especially loved Bonaventure. When his daughter Gracie was young, the two walked around its grounds for hours, every day. For several years before he was diagnosed, Jack's health began to deteriorate. During that time, he began photographing hundreds of stone angels around Bonaventure and other cemeteries. "I believe he was unknowingly trying to reclaim his spiritual tradition," Susan said.

In the months before I was diagnosed, Linda began observing that I was restless, sleepless, irritable. "You weren't yourself," she later said. Jack's family noticed a similar pattern, and it colored his work. For the first time, he began to forgo the hyperfocused style that had been his trademark and started taking blurry, unfocused images—especially of water.

"Jack never did anything that was unintentional," Susan said. "And his most deeply personal work was always focused on water. He had this reoccurring dream that he was somewhere photographing, that he wouldn't be paying attention, and suddenly he would realize that the tide had come in and washed all his camera equipment out to sea."

What did it mean?

"As an artist, I think he feared that his work wouldn't be remembered," she said. "But the peace he got to around his dying is that while your camera may have washed out to sea, while you were busy creating the art, the art was creating you. And you are left with this amazing life that you participated in.

"When Jack was dying," she continued, "he would ask me to sing him a lullaby I often sang to the girls when they were little. It was a song about the river and how it carries us home. The night before he died, I fell asleep briefly lying next to him and was instructed in a dream to tell him that dying was like floating in a boat on the river. He was just to relax and let it carry him. Afterward, I found a box of Polaroids next to his bed, containing all the last images he shot. On top was a blurred photograph of a canoe, sitting on a dock, alongside a river."

———

THE FEILER FAMILY PLOT is located at Lot 570, Section Q, just off Nunez Way. It's shaped like an oblong trapezoid, sixteen by eleven paces, and is lined with a low granite coping wall. Two live oaks grow on either side, their trunks speckled with lichen. Some mushrooms poke up from the ground.

The six existing graves are spread along the back. My grandfather had asked that his tombstone be engraved "HE DID WHAT HE WAS SUPPOSED TO DO," but after his suicide, my parents decided that epitaph would be inappropriate. His stone now reads "BELOVED HUSBAND AND FATHER."

I quickly tallied the ages of the deceased—sixty-one, sixty-two, seventy-seven, seventy-eight, eighty-two, eighty-nine. Forty-four seemed gulpingly young.

A stone bench sits in a corner with the inscription "MAY THE BEAUTY OF THEIR LIVES SHINE FOREVER / MAY OUR LIVES ALWAYS BRING HONOR TO THEIR MEMORY." I sat down to take in the scene.

The afternoon light was just sieving through the trees. I could just glimpse the Wilmington River and beyond it the bridge toward Tybee. A hawk circled overhead. John Muir had observed bald eagles roosting in the live oaks; today those same trees were buzzing with cicadas.

Linda arrived a few minutes later and joined me on the bench. A few weeks before I learned that I had cancer, I finally got around to updating my will. At the time, I asked Linda where she thought we should be buried. She chose Bonaventure. We were married in Savannah, she said; our girls would come here their entire lives. This sandy soil was our touchstone.

Today was her first visit to this spot.

"It's so beautiful," she said, slipping her arm around my back.

"It reminds me of a line from Genesis," I said. "After each day of Creation, God looks at the sky, the water, and the land, and announces that it is 'good.' This place is good."

I kept scanning the ground, imagining where my parents would someday rest, as well as Linda and me. But I couldn't settle on one spot. It was like a nightmare in which you are about to die but wake just before the decisive moment.

Thunder clapped, and we looked up at the sky. Ominous charcoal clouds had swept in quickly over the marsh in the familiar choreography of coastal afternoons. Soon, thick dollops of rain were piercing the canopy of leaves. Within seconds, we were caught in a downpour.

We stood up to go. As we did, I began reciting the words from my favorite poem, Shel Silverstein's "This Bridge," which I had long ago asked Linda to read at my funeral. It tells of a road that leads around the world, through Gypsy camps and spicy Arab fairs, through wondrous woods where unicorns run free. It ends with a searing image.

But this bridge will only take you halfway there—
The last few steps you'll have to take alone.

Just as I finished, Linda pressed her lips to mine. "You don't have to say that," she whispered. "You're going to be here for a long, long time." Tears were streaming down our cheeks, salt trickling into our mouths. The rain was matting our hair. My crutches tumbled to the ground. And in the darkened cathedral of a Bonaventure thundershower, we clung to each other, pressed our foreheads together, and kissed on the land where we would one day rest forever.

19

CHRONICLES OF THE LOST YEAR

volume VI

April 14

Dear Friends and Family,

The cheery clarion of sun wakes us up most mornings
these days and lingers well past dinnertime, though
chilly showers still puddle the ground and keep our
coats and mittens close by. But the pear tree across the
street has just erupted into full blossom, our own private
promise that spring is here to enliven us again.

Those blossoms have come to signal another yearly
milestone for me. Four years ago tonight, Linda and I
ventured outside from our apartment in Manhattan.
Then, as now, we mazed our way through a protracted,

nine-month ordeal, full of doctors' offices, endless tests, and the occasional outburst of anxiety. Then, as now, one of us was just being allowed up from three months in bed with the occasional foray onto the couch. And then, as now, we had counted the minutes until the arrival of spring. That night we sat in a neighborhood Italian restaurant, ordered flatbread pizza and our first glass of wine in months, and simply enjoyed being out of the house. What I most remember from that evening was looking into Linda's eyes and thinking, "She's ready."

It was April 14, 2005. The next day she would give birth to our daughters.

We tell time around our house by the girls' birthday (and trust me: it comes up hourly, no matter the season!), and this year is no different. After nine and a half months, twenty-nine nights in the hospital, one hundred visits to the doctor, a thousand pills, and several thirty-pound swings of weight, my chemotherapy has come to an end. I'm done. As promised, the last several rounds were challenging, as my body got weaker and the cumulative side effects worse. The short-term pain in my leg became intense with each dosage. And by the end, as I waited for the results of the final blood test that would either send me back into the hospital or absolve me from any more visits to the clinic, I was holding my breath. "Your numbers are great," the nurse reported in a call. "You

don't have to come tomorrow." I put down the receiver
and broke down on the couch.

I arrived at this day with some trepidation. On the one
hand, the daily assault on my body that began last July
has finally ended. On the other hand, we are no longer
actively attacking the problem. We have given my body
the best treatment it can receive, and we have either
killed the cancer cells that were likely circulating in my
blood, or we have not. And we have no way of knowing.
(For this reason I will get multiple scans every four
months for the foreseeable future.) In the final weeks I
begged my doctors to give me more chemotherapy if they
thought it would help. The kids, who more commonly
get this disease, are given more. But my doctors felt
the possible benefits did not outweigh the considerable
downsides and declared me finished. Suddenly time,
which since last summer had been completely dictated
by the relentless schedule of treatment, would become
my own again, both a welcome and an unnerving
development.

With the few weeks that have passed, my appetite, my
energy, and even my hair have begun to return. (I had an
inkling of hair in January, but like those sucker February
daffodils that are wiped out by late-season snow, my
fuzz quickly got its comeuppance. I am disheartened to
report that my hair seems to be returning with bald spots

in place, a cruel *Groundhog Day* curse to relive the arrival of middle age.) And in perhaps the most vivid parallel with pregnancy, my mind has already begun to erase the unpleasant memories. So before my own brainwashing is complete, let me close this chapter of my Lost Year by saying what I said to Linda that final night of chemo: "May you live to a ripe old age, kiss good night the ones you love, and die peacefully in your sleep, rather than go through what I just went through."

One unabashedly positive outcome of the end of chemo is that the full healing of my surgically repaired leg, which was impeded by the chemotherapy, can finally begin. As Dr. Healey said to me recently, "The clock starts now." The reason is that until the bone fully fuses with the prosthesis, I must remain on crutches and limit the weight I put on my left leg. Nearly four months after my surgery, I am making considerable progress with my mobility. I now stand in the shower, bend over to put on my shoes and socks, and take short, crutch-aided walks in the neighborhood. Many times I look down at my leg and feel it's a miracle it's still there.

But there are other times when I am nearly overwhelmed by the deadweight I am dragging around and the long road I have to endure. The big picture is that one needs three muscles to walk—the calf, hamstring, and glutes— and all of mine are basically fine. I have three principal problems: limited flexibility in my ankle; restricted bending of my knee; and the loss of one-third of my quad. These alternately make sitting, walking, sleeping, driving, and making peanut-butter-and-jelly sandwiches challenging. (My wife reports that I somehow have enough mobility to remove dishes from the cupboard but not enough to place them in the dishwasher.)

I have begun physical therapy, and my team is bullish on my recovery. Last week I was on an exercise bike; yesterday I was walking in a pool. But the process—call it phase four of our war—will extend for at least a year. I've been joking that physical therapy means taking it one grunt at a time. Or, as Dr. Healey vividly said of the chorus of aarghs and ughs that comprise a normal session, "In PT, we measure progress in decibels."

But how about those birthday girls? How are they doing? Back in January I lay awake one night feeling that my protracted stay in the hospital following surgery and subsequent bed rest at home had left me somewhat estranged from the girls. Today, after three straight months around the house and over a month of crutching up and down the stairs, those memories seem happily remote. Tybee and Eden are barreling into their fourth birthday (or maybe I should say careening on their brand-new "big-girl bikes" with training wheels) as feisty, sensitive, cheery, talkative, and imaginative little preteens—oops, little girls. They have weathered an enormous amount of irregularity in recent months, and they have done so with grace and good humor.

I am pleased to report that their color palette has tiptoed beyond purple and pink—Eden has added blue and green; Tybee has added chocolate. Ballet has been augmented with swimming. The washing of hair and the brushing of teeth now often pass without U.N. intervention. But their minds most ignite and their giggles most endear when they are making up fantasy games with their imaginary friends, spontaneously inventing verses to a song, or chuckling through a rhyming game at dinner. I knew I had to recalibrate my view of them when I recently found myself talking about "Terrific Tuesdays" and "Wonderful Wednesdays." "What kind of words are those?" Tybee asked. "They're a kind of rhyme," I said. "But rhymes sound the same," Eden corrected me. I gulped, saw my future flash before my eyes, and proceeded to explain the meaning of "alliteration" . . . to three-year-olds! I, of course, had to look up how to spell it, but by the next day they no longer did. Eden and Tybee may not yet have to do homework, but we do, just to keep up with them!

And yes, there are differences between the two. Eden is the bolder dancer, the boundary tester, and the seeker of the spotlight. Tybee is the speedier reader, the more beauty conscious, and the melodramatic singer-songwriter. Tybee also appears to be the Internationalist of the two, snarfing up all the German and French books she can get her hands on and insisting that Linda teach her Hindi after a recent stint in India. Eden, by contrast, is the America Firster. Recently Tybee was quizzing me about why I say "I love you" so much. "It's the special language of daddies," I said. "Would you like to know how to count to ten in 'Daddy'?" Then I began to say, " 'I love you. I love you. I love you . . .' " all the way up to ten. Not missing a beat, Tybee announced, "Do you know how to count to ten in 'Tybee'?" Then off she went on her own string of "I love you's." Eden was having none of it. "Would you like to know how to count to ten in 'Eden'?" she asked. "One. Two. Three. Four . . ."

Above all, if you had told me last summer we could get through the brunt of my treatment with only a handful of awkward moments with the girls, I would have wept at the chance. Today, I see that they may even have learned how to be a bit more sensitive, an ounce more caring, a dose more compassionate, as a result of their experience with me. They run to embrace the girl with an amputated leg on the playground. They spot the rabbit with the crutches tucked away in the back of the children's book illustration. They promise to take care of each other the minute one manifests even the slightest sniffle and have invented a special cheer to make any medicine they must take go down.

A month or so ago I made my first outing with the girls
since the surgery in late December. Linda's mom and
I took them for pizza a few blocks away. After dinner,
the girls were holding Grandma DeeDee's hands as we
rounded the corner for home. I was bringing up the
rear, a block behind, when Tybee suddenly broke away
from her grandmother, came sprinting back to me, and
offered to help with my crutches. "I love you, Daddy," she
said. A few days later Eden woke up in the middle of the
night and came to my side of the bed and told me about
some monster or nightmare or little girl fright. She came
into my arms for a cuddle, and then I persuaded her to
let me walk her back to her room. As I got out of bed,
she reached to hand me my crutches. If I could cling to
one memory from this last year, it would be me and my
daughter, walking down a darkened hall a little after
four in the morning, with five little fingers grasping
the spongy handle underneath my hand. The crutch at
that moment melted from my arm, as it was supporting
her instead. I, of course, didn't need it anymore. I was
walking on air.

Us. I mentioned earlier that we tell time by the girlies'
birthday. What I meant was that for Linda and me, April
15 has always been not just about them, but about us, too.
That first year it was about Linda making it through the
shoals of a high-risk pregnancy, enduring the setbacks
of bed rest, and prevailing through the ordeal of giving

birth to two six-pound babies within thirty-two minutes
of each other. Then it became about surviving our own
ineptitude and maneuvering through the Herculean
challenges of taking care of two babies when we didn't
know how to take care of one—and still managing to
emerge speaking to each other. Then it became about the
weaning, the potty training, the picky eating—the toddler
two-step of terribles and tantrums that we had to traverse
in tandem.

And then came this year.

And we made it through that, too.

When Linda was pregnant, every night before going to
sleep we had a little poem we would recite to the girls. We
both had lines; I'll put Linda's lines in italics.

> Daddy loves you.
> Daddy loves your Mommy.
> *Your Mommy loves your Daddy.*
> Your Mommy loves you.
> You love each other.
> *But . . .*
> You're still individuals.
> *You're still individuals.*

Then we added a kind of countdown clock—our way of

encouraging them to stay in Mommy's tummy for thirty-six weeks, full term for twins.

> You've been in Mommy's tummy twenty-four
> weeks . . .
> *Stay in Mommy's tummy twelve more weeks!*

This poem became so meaningful that it was the first thing I uttered to Tybee and Eden on the night they were born—my attempt to calm their tears and dim the din as they made their way into an unfamiliar world. For months afterward, when we put the girls to bed, we repeated our poem and reversed our ticking clock, beginning to log time upward. Nowadays, we recite this poem only once a year, on their birthday, and we will do so again tomorrow night before they go to sleep. They will probably ignore us, or beseech us to read another real poem, or begin the nightly delaying tactics: "Mommy, you forgot my water." "Daddy, will you sit with us for a few minutes?" "Is tomorrow a skirt day or a dress day?" But we will persevere, put our arms around each other, and start crying before we reach the end.

Because this birthday marks another singular time. These days, when we catch each other's eye as we dart between some ringing phone and some overboiling pot, when one of our daughters says the most absurd, charming thing, when we hear that lullaby that once drove us batty but now makes us nostalgic, or when one of our arms reaches across the bed in the middle of the night and strokes a shoulder or patch of skin, for the first time in what seems like a very long time, we don't think only of losing each other. We allow ourselves the flicker of a thought that maybe we have endured the worst. Maybe we'll get another year. Or maybe many more.

So on what is widely regarded as one of the most dreaded days in America—April 15—we hope you'll take a moment and smile at this special milestone for us, be a crutch for someone you know who may be hurting, and reach out an arm to someone you love and mark the simple miracle of another year.

And sometime this spring, when a tree near you is blossoming, please, take a walk for me.

Love,

Bruce

20

JOSHUA

Harvest Miracles

THE SKY OVER THE RIO Grande valley in northern New Mexico is wide and round. The striations of clouds that hover over the gorge reach so far to the left and right they seem to arc around the horizon like two arms about to embrace you. The fullness of color at dusk—peach, almond, pink—reminds me of the paintings my four-year-olds have just begun making in which the paint no longer puddles alone in the middle of the paper but spreads to the edge of the sheet. The view here bleeds off the page.

"The sunsets in New Mexico are like no place on earth," says Joshua Ramo, who should know. A native of Albuquerque, the itinerant author, business consultant, and stunt pilot has seen the sun go down in Beijing, London, Kyoto, Rome, and Provence—and that's just in the last month. "Twilight here is a spectator sport. People pull over in their cars to watch the sun go down."

We are sitting in a field of wildflowers on the side of Lama Mountain, a spiritual retreat in the Carson National Forest, 8,600 feet above sea level. A wildfire raced through here a decade ago. A knee-high brush of sage, lavender, bluebells, columbine, and pink nodding onion has sprouted up to cover the ground, but the sky is still scarred by barkless Ponderosa pines. The spirit of renewal is manifest here, but you cannot take in the scenery without being reminded of the ever presence of grief.

Joshua is the newest of my friends and the last of my dads, and he has brought me here on a summer's retreat to purge me of my chemo, mark the boundary of my treatment, and distill the essence of his advice to our girls.

But there was a catch: First we had to spend a day meditating, fasting, and not speaking.

"You mean you brought me halfway across the country to talk with you for two days only to then *not* talk to you for a day?" I asked.

"That's the Ramo way!" he said.

That's the Ramo paradox.

WHEN I FIRST THOUGHT of the Council of Dads, I envisioned a group of names on a list. The dads were individuals who would have their own private relationships with the girls. But as I started to share the idea with the men, the Council began to evolve. For starters, the dads took action. One sent a magazine subscription; another stopped by more frequently; a third asked for more photos of the girls. As one of them said, "I think it's part of my responsibility as a Council member to know the girls as they grow up."

Even more surprising, the men took a keen interest in one another—with equal parts curiosity, kinship, and rivalry. A fraternity developed. And suddenly my notion of a list no longer applied. It was more like a community, a circle, a Stonehenge assembly where the girls could seek relief.

In this circle I had certain figures: my childhood buddy, my camp counselor, my college roommate, my business partner, my closest confidant. But I had one last hole to fill.

"It's your creative side," Linda said. "The part of you that's visual, that photographs, that brings back masks and Bedouin carpets from your travels. You see things in color, not black and white. When the girls ask me why we have a Japanese kimono on the wall, or why your favorite color was orange, I need someone to explain how you looked at the world."

Joshua is that person.

He is the man who looks around the room and, while everyone else is sizing up one another, says, "Hey, isn't this beautiful!?" He's the little brother of the group, the one who lives by his own schedule, whose hair is a little unruly and who shows up for Thanksgiving with a beard just when Mom thinks he's finally cleaned himself up. He's the maverick, who stares into space instead of doing his homework and who quotes the obscure poet or rock lyric and believes they're really true. He's the one who still says "dude" without irony.

And he's the one the girls all choose because they find him charming.

I first met Joshua six years earlier at a conference on a mountaintop in Utah. A onetime foreign editor at *Time* magazine, Joshua knew Linda through their shared interest in international affairs. At the time, he was living in Beijing, immersing himself in the study of Chinese. In the next few years, he would rise to become a top China analyst—writing papers, consulting for Fortune 500 CEOs, and eventually offering commentary alongside Bob Costas at the opening ceremonies of the Beijing Olympics.

With his rock-star pout and rock-climber's body, Joshua was known to make attendees at international confabs swoon. With his economist's mind and poet's soul, he was known to intrigue clients with his Zen-like pronouncements. He looked like a cross between James Dean and Steve Jobs.

He was also a confirmed—and even delighted— bachelor. That night in Utah we fell into a late-night conversation about God, his restless ambitions, and a certain girl from Tibet. When our conversation ended around 3:00 A.M., I went back to my room; he went to the hot tub. For years, Joshua stopped by occasionally when he passed through New York, but Linda and I were up to our ears in sippy cups and diapers.

Then I got sick, and overnight Joshua became a fixture in our lives, a monthly comet and comforting compatriot. It was during those months that I discovered a new side of him—a side that reminded me of, well, me. He was the man in the bespoke suit who donned a bomber jacket and barnstormed around Namibia in a borrowed plane. He was the hard-driving jet-setter who also volunteered at an AIDS hospice in South Africa. He was the man who loved beauty but was also drawn to pain.

In my year of gray, he helped restore my love of color.

Even as my body suffered, he reminded me to keep my eyes clear.

Linda was moved. "Few people this year were more attuned to your joy and suffering," she said. "If the girls wanted to know how deeply you feel things and how vividly you view the world, I would send them to him."

It was that sensitivity I wanted Joshua to convey to our girls. He is the one who would teach them how to appreciate the perfect panorama or the exquisite view. He's the person who would explain that even when they hurt, they should still find time for wonder. He's the man who would show the girls how to marvel at the everyday miracles around them.

Joshua would teach them how to see.

———

"WHY ARE WE HERE?" I asked.

The requisite silence and hunger had accumulated, and we were sitting the next day by a bubbling stream in a cluster of quaking aspens.

Joshua was silent for a full minute.

"We're here to talk about fatherhood, and in many ways New Mexico is my father," he said. "The role a father plays in a boy's life is to make him a man and to show him how to see the world. My own father is a wonderful man. He's one of my closest friends. Whenever I have an important decision to make, he's the person I call at the very end for advice. But when I was growing up I needed something different."

He gestured toward the sanctuary around us. "The New Mexico wilderness is what made me who I am today. It imbued me with a love of beauty. It taught me how to take risks. It showed me how to push myself."

"So when you look out at this landscape, what do you see?"

"What I see is a constant unfolding visual poem," he said. "This stream, the clouds, the sunset last night. And when you grow up learning to see like that, you never stop."

I asked him how he would teach someone else to see that way.

"It has very little to do with what you are looking at," he said, "and everything to do with who you are. Seeing that way requires a certain internal stillness. The best aerobatic pilots fly their planes without any reference to what's going on outside the cockpit. They don't need to look at the horizon; they don't need to see the ground. They look inside themselves for a sense of direction that's more accurate—but harder to cultivate."

Joshua grew up wanting to be a pilot but abandoned his dream for journalism. Within a decade he was a paragon of the mainstream media at a time when the mainstream media still had clout. Then, in 2000, while on assignment in the Democratic Republic of Congo, he witnessed a massacre. "I basically decided that I was seeing things that were so awful, that just being a journalist wasn't going to be enough for me." He left the profession. The man of words would try to become a man of action.

"My favorite quote comes from the Roman general Epaminondas," Joshua said. "In A.D. 70, he was rallying his troops for battle one day, when he sat on a chair and it collapsed underneath him. His men freaked out. It was a horrible omen. But Epaminondas stood up and announced, 'This is a sign that we must be up and doing.'"

He went on. "What I love about this line is that

it shows the importance of how you see a particular event. You can turn a bad omen into a good one. Also, it endorses the power of an active life. Especially these days when around any corner could be a war, an epidemic, or some other unexpected crisis, being active is what the world demands of us."

———

A FEW DAYS BEFORE I left for New Mexico, Linda and I were trapped with the girls on an airport tarmac while wave after wave of thundershowers passed overhead. The thirty or so passengers on our plane were growing increasingly agitated.

An hour later, the rain stopped, the clouds parted, and the most idyllic rainbow appeared in the sky. Tybee was the first to see it. "Eden, look! A rainbow!" she cried. "Where!?" Eden asked. "Oh, Daddy, *look*! Our first rainbow! It's so beautiful, I can hardly STAND it!!" The two of them then proceeded to dance on their seats with pure, unbridled glee. It was as if a unicorn had swept down from the clouds, plucked a mermaid from the seas, and were waltzing alongside our window.

And the entire plane full of passengers, upon seeing their joy, burst into applause.

I told Joshua that story as we were sitting by the stream. "That's what I'm talking about," he said. "The world is ceaselessly filled with miracles like that rainbow. Sometimes it just takes a crappy situation to force us to see differently." He added. "That's what happened when you got sick."

I asked him why cancer had been such a boon to our friendship.

"My first thought when you got sick is that you can't have enough people around you at a time like that. Just jump in with an extra set of hands. But then you started showing me how to deal with a moment in which beauty wasn't unspooling every day, but in which something ugly was happening. Yet you dealt with it with a grace and humor that I don't think I could have brought to it, frankly. I would like to say it was a big selfless thing for me to be with you, but the reality was it was an education about what humans are capable of."

"If the girls came to you and asked what it was like during this year, what would you tell them?"

"I would tell them I saw a man who had lived his life in such a way that when he was confronted with the worst possible thing that can face a man, he was able to face it with no regrets. Think of how few people can say that. I've been with other people who are struggling through potentially terminal disease. I know what that looks like. You didn't look like that. And the reason, I think, is that you know who you are. You have a clear sense of internal navigation."

"So how do you teach someone that? If my girls asked you for help in discovering themselves, what would you do?"

"Ah, that's easy," he said. "I believe the best teacher

is beauty. I'll teach them to memorize Auden poems and Shakespeare sonnets so that wherever they are at any given moment in the world, they can just sit under a tree and have Auden or Shakespeare or whomever as their companion for an afternoon. I'll give them the sound of Mahler symphonies that they can hear again and again and that will always trigger similar emotions. I'll show them how to appreciate Chinese calligraphy, which is an expression of your internal energy. If you have any doubt in your heart, it shows up in the brushstroke."

Joshua had taken off his shoes and was running his feet through the water. The spring that had barely gurgled when we arrived had slowly gained strength and filled the basin in front of us. The next morning we would drive down from the mountain and have dinner with his mom and dad. Soon, the confirmed bachelor would start talking about getting married and becoming a father himself. Peter Pan was growing up, while retaining his ability to see like a child.

"What I want Eden and Tybee to know," he continued, "is how easy it is to see beauty. How the wonder they felt on that plane never has to leave them. Miracles are all around them. They just have to learn to see through the clouds, and go out and harvest those miracles themselves. And, of course, I'd want them to know that this way of seeing never left you, even when you were sick. And it's how all of us who love them want them to see the world, too."

21

ALWAYS LEARN TO JUGGLE
ON THE SIDE OF A HILL

JOHN HEALEY HAS A PRINT of Fenway Park hanging above his desk. It shows a boy's-eye view of the
playing field, with Old Glory flapping up above, sky
the color of Superman's tights, and the Green Monster
looming overhead. To the right of the print is a photograph of Carl Yastrzemski's final at bat on October 2,
1983. To the left is a Red Sox calendar, turned to the previous October, nine months earlier.

"As you can see, baseball is my first love," said Dr.
Healey, who grew up outside Boston.

So when I asked him how he learned to juggle, I
should not have been surprised when he came back to
the most storied Red Stocking of all.

"I played baseball in high school," he said, "but my

coach told the baseball people at Yale that I wasn't good enough to play for them. In the freshman league at college, however, I led the team in batting. I actually hit .406, which is the famous average of my favorite player, Ted Williams, the last .400 hitter in baseball."

With no slots left on the varsity squad, the coach invited the sophomore prodigy to be a player-grunt, which allowed him to practice, but obliged him to handle tedious logistics, like renting the bus for out-of-town games. "I had ten at bats that year," Dr. Healey recalled. "I mostly sat on the bench. In those days, some people chewed tobacco to pass the time. I learned to juggle."

The attraction, he said, was the arc of the ball. "It all came back to my favorite geometric shape, which is a parabola. Watching a long fly ball, or foul tip to the catcher, is beautiful to me. It has an extremely calming effect, like a piece of clothing you buy that is immediately comfortable. That was the appeal of juggling. It's three parabolas at once!"

"Wait. You have a favorite geometric shape?" I asked.

"Absolutely. I know the mathematical formula. Also, there's a spinning of the object that's not visible at a distance that I find fascinating."

When his roommate came up with the idea to design Yale's first-ever mascot costume—a bulldog with a giant head—Dr. Healey put on the outfit for several football games a year. America's leading orthopedic cancer surgeon was Yale's first juggling mascot. And when his friend later tried out for Ringling Brothers' Clown College, Dr. Healey tagged along and auditioned on a whim. He was turned down.

Thirty-five years later, was juggling still relevant to his life?

"Sure. On a concrete level, I still love going to baseball games and seeing long fly balls or pop-ups. Some are easy to catch, what are referred to as cans of corn; others are extremely challenging.

"And in a more metaphoric sense," he continued, "this is how I view my life. The easy ones are easy and anybody could catch those. It's the hard ones, the ones with the little extra spin, that really distinguish a pro. One of my goals is to try and reduce that extra spin and turn it into a can of corn. That's the constant challenge of my work. I turn the obstacles into something manageable. I take comfort in saying, 'I know how to do this.'"

JOHN HEALEY KNOWS HOW to do a lot of things. The walls in his office not covered in Red Sox memorabilia brim with citations, degrees, certificates of appreciation, a profile from *New York* magazine's "Best Doctors" issue, and a giant *Time* magazine cover, "Hope in the War Against Cancer." His résumé overflows with over 250 articles, 40 chapters in books, and 5 patents. He's a member of Alpha Omega Alpha, the medical honor society, and serves as president of the International Society of Limb Salvage, perhaps the least euphemistic name I've ever heard.

But none of these are what make him compelling. That accrues to the bow ties with Santas and candy canes, the Doughboy grin and unexpected laugh, the string of wise expressions that would make my dad proud: *I hate your cancer almost as much as you do; This is a war and I intend to win it; Things like this change you, usually for the better.*

Above all, it's the way he delivers these lines, with the long pause before responding to each question that makes you wonder whether you just inadvertently called his mother a harlot; the snail-like parceling out of words; the idiosyncratic aura that makes him seem like a character out of a Harry Potter novel. He even has a name J. K. Rowling couldn't improve. What would *you* call the prestidigitatorial Dumbledore who can cure the uncurable and salvage the unsalvageable? How about . . . *Healey!*

It was these quirks—and the erudition behind them—that drew me to see him on the anniversary of my diagnosis to garner counsel for myself, and for my girls. Before my "Lost Year" ended, I needed to hear from him. In my year of fathers, he was my father figure.

I began by asking him why he does what he does.

"I have a love for it," he said. "It's a blessing that I can take that love and fulfill what I feel is a personal obligation to use my God-given talents to make the world a better place. I found something I am not only good at, but, at the risk of being prideful, I strive to be *the* best in the world at. In fact, every day when I wake up and look in the mirror while I'm shaving, I say, 'Today I am going to be *The Best Doctor in the World.*' It's something that I haven't achieved but continue to strive for."

"At every step along the way," I said, "first medical school, then orthopedics, then cancer, you chose something narrower, darker, bleaker."

He nodded ruefully. "I had broken seven different bones at seven different times," he said, "playing sports and thinking that I was bigger and stronger and better than I was. But I overcame these injuries and went back on the field. So my initial instinct was to be a sports medicine doctor.

"But I soon found that taking care of people who want to play tennis that weekend wasn't sufficiently satisfying to me. That's important. I'm glad someone's doing that. But I gravitated to where the most interesting questions were. Cancer, as the biggest horizon, the toughest problem, and the greatest need, was the logical choice."

"But that means a lot of your patients don't get better."

"There are no greater successes and no greater failures," he said. "So you have to have an ability to deal with that. If you get to the point where you stop feeling it, then you're not doing your job. But if you feel it too much, it paralyzes you. It's defining courage not as blindly going into a dangerous situation, but really understanding how dangerous it's going to be, yet somehow mustering the courage to go.

"Paraphrasing Patton," he continued, " 'War brings out the best in people.' Sure, the worst. But also, the best. And since this is the greatest war in my discipline, I get to glimpse into the heart, the spirit, and the mind of people who have to deal with this enormous challenge and see how they find the strength they didn't believe they had. Even their mother didn't think they had it. But they do. And they show me how great humanity and the human condition can be."

He paused.

"So even in the failures," Dr. Healey said, "I glimpse greatness. In fact, the greatest people I know are people who have survived this disease. They have a clarity about life and what they want to accomplish that is mind-blowing. It's a privilege to be their doctor."

"You told us in our first meeting that most people who go through this experience are changed," I said, "usually for the better. What does that mean?"

"They understand themselves better. They are less distracted by the transient, unimportant things. Family becomes more central. Plus, they usually develop a constructive spirituality, one not based on dogma but real-life experience. And they are more sensitive to the suffering of others. They have an empathy that is part of the greatness of human beings."

"So here is the question anybody would ask," I said.

" 'How do I get me some of that without going through this?' " I gestured toward my leg.

"I guess that's what I'm doing," Dr. Healey said. "I'm getting some of it. It's true for me, and I believe it's a widespread truth, that those of us in the healing professions want to believe that if we do good works, we're not going to get sick. Of course that's nonsense, but we like to believe it.

"But in the process, we do gain vicariously from treating others. I know for myself, having access to the Full Monty of human emotions helps me enormously in my own life. So what I would say is, 'Engage those who have problems. Understand their situation. Mostly, just listen.' As my father used to say, 'You don't learn anything when your mouth is open. Your ears, that's a different story . . .' "

———

I DIDN'T LEARN TO juggle in college. I learned in summer camp, when I was thirteen. My counselor had studied under the legendary mime Marcel Marceau and taught us various tricks, like touching a window that wasn't there or playing tug-of-war with an imaginary rope. One morning he set out to teach us how to juggle. We purloined oranges from the breakfast room, stood on the gravel hill outside our tent, and bumbled our way from single toss, to double, to three-orb cascade.

There was only one problem: We were learning with

fruit at the precipice of a slope, which meant every time we dropped an orange (which was hundreds of times in those early hours) our little spheres of stolen sunshine would drop to the ground, pulpify, then wobble to the bottom of the incline, leaving us covered in rind, dripping in juice, and exhausted from scurrying after them. It was a fool's errand, like the clown who refuses to see how half-witted he is.

Except it worked.

And forever after, that ill-conceived experiment became something of a life motto for me: Always learn to juggle on the side of a hill. If you're going to try something, try it. If you're going to make the pose, a director friend of mine liked to say, make the pose. Don't half commit.

And whether it was our shared heritage as teenage cutups, or my need to see my doctor as a savior, I came to view Dr. Healey as the embodiment of this ideal. *This is a war and I intend to win it. I'm going to be the last man standing. Today I'm going to be the best doctor in the world.*

He lived his life on the side of a hill.

Given that outlook, I wondered what lessons he might draw from my case, especially if I turned out to be one of his failures.

"It's fifteen years from now," I said. "One of my daughters comes to you and says, 'Why did my daddy die?' What would you tell her?"

The master of pauses paused far longer than I had ever witnessed. Then he cleared his throat. Then he leaned forward.

"I would say that there is no simple answer to that," he said. "On one hand, everybody dies. Many people actually never live, and your daddy lived. It was just not as long as any of us would have liked. But he lived well, and he provided a great example for you. And as sad as it is that he's not here, you can take some solace in knowing how much he loved you and how hard he fought to be here for you."

"So she says to you, 'You've been around many who died. How should I live?'"

Again he thought for a minute. "Have a joy in everything you do," he said. "Help those around you. Make a mark on this world."

"'And if along the way,' she says, 'I end up in your office, or one like it, with some condition, what do I need to fight my own war?'"

Here the pauses finally waned. Dr. Healey was filling with purpose. He was that warrior, who first looked me in the eye a year earlier and said, "Give me your hand. I'll show you how to do this. We're going to do this together." And in that instant, when my legs were most bowed and my eyes most frightened, I would have followed him anywhere he led.

"I would say to your daughter, 'Do your homework,'" Dr. Healey said. "'Get the best allies you can, both medically and personally. Remain focused on the goal. And don't look back, because that just squanders your energy, disrupts your focus, and sows seeds of doubt and recrimination that are destructive for yourself and the people around you.'

"It's what I call the Satchel Paige approach," he said. "Satchel being maybe the greatest pitcher of all time, but being a black man, he was barred from the Major Leagues. After Jackie Robinson, he was pitching for the Cleveland Indians, and, at age forty-two, had finally made the All-Star Team. A reporter asked him, 'Hey, Satch, don't you regret not being up in your prime?' And Satchel responded, 'Don't look back. Something might be gaining on you.'

"I think that very much applies to cancer, to medical situations, and to all aspects of life. You need to learn from history but don't dwell on it. You need to educate yourself, but don't get mired in it. Look to the future. That's what your father would want you to do, I would tell your girls, because that's what he did himself."

22

CHRONICLES OF THE LOST YEAR

volume VII

July 13

Dear Friends and Family,

The morning sun is shimmering off Snug Harbor this week, and the skies over Cape Cod are as bountiful as the blueberries our girls picked this morning. The clear days and fresh fields are a welcome relief from a long spell in New York marked by "May Gray," "June Gloom," and this year's Summer Solstice, the Cloudiest Day of the Year.

Last week I went to visit a friend I hadn't seen in a while. I sat in his chair in New York's trendy Meatpacking District surrounded by disco balls, leopard divans, and dolls with pink hair. Michael Angelo (yes, that's his real name) gave me a hug as we talked about the horrendous ordeal that has elapsed since we last met. Then he went to work. It was 5:30 P.M. on the 365th day of my Lost Year, and I was about to do something I had not done in that entire time.

I was getting my hair cut.

Twelve months have passed since I first learned I had an osteosarcoma in my left femur. During my recent quarterly checkups, I received much good news. There are no signs of cancer in my bones or lungs. My prosthesis is growing nicely into my femur. As Dr. Healey said, "You are on your way to recovery. Truly."

He then added, "But we both know . . ."

On the sobering front, the chemotherapy has left me with neuropathy in the tips of several fingers. The fibular graft is not fusing to my femur in quite the way we hoped, and I may have to have more surgery to correct it. And my leg is still a burden. We reach this one-year milestone with relief, if not champagne. My Lost Year is over, but my long road continues.

Since April, I have been attending a superb physical therapy facility at the Hospital for Special Surgery in Manhattan. (Its official name, still visible on the

uniforms of its employees, is The Hospital for the
Ruptured and Crippled. Branding by Dickens?) I am
under the sage, demanding care of Theresa Chiaia, a
onetime basketball prodigy who now regularly supervises
the care of assorted Mets, Yankees, and other area divas.
On my first visit, she carefully analyzed every stretch,
bend, and lift of my leg, then announced, "I think your
prospects are promising."

Theresa has me on a strict schedule of exercises, weights,
and stationary bike riding. I also work out in a pool and
walk on an AquaCiser, which is basically a treadmill with
shoulder-high glass walls that fill with water. It's like
strolling in a washing machine.

The encouraging news is that I am making measurable
progress, occasionally walk with only one crutch, and
hope to move to a cane by fall. But the truth is that
after fifty-two straight weeks on crutches (that's nearing
three percent of my life), I sometimes grow weary of the
challenge.

Having said that, people often remark that they hope to
live long enough to take advantage of a medical miracle. I
have lived that long. Twenty years ago doctors would have
cut off my leg; even a decade ago, my surgery would not
have been possible. That I stand today—and on two legs,
no less—is a testament to the skill and tenderness of a

great many well-trained hands and minds. Whatever life
I enjoy from now on comes entirely from their grace, and
for that we will always be grateful.

So how are the girls? Great. Now that the Fourth of July has
passed, I think we can say with some confidence that
Eden and Tybee's April 15 birthday has finally come
to an end. Their final gift was a week in California,
during which they visited LEGOLAND, made their
own dresses in Beverly Hills, and squeezed hand-picked
lemons for their first lemonade stand. Their mother,
the guru of entrepreneurship, was pleased with their
marketing acumen and their monopolistic control of
the playground but was concerned that they underpriced
their product, charging only a dime instead of a quarter.
One thing they definitely learned: Don't dump your till
in the sandbox!

As time came to leave Los Angeles, Tybee announced,
"I never want to go back to Brooklyn." Some of this was
surely the hospitality we received, but more, we suspect,
came from having the undivided attention of her parents.
Tybee and Eden are growing up quickly these days. They
enjoy running their fingers through my hair and are
showing few signs of the trauma they endured. Above all,
they appreciate having Daddy back.

Recently, during our nightly game of Bad & Good,

Eden's good was, "Daddy is using one crutch now, so I can hold his hand." Tybee followed with this bit of wisdom: "I have so much love in my body for you, Daddy, that I can't stop giving you hugs and kisses. And when I have no more love left, I just drink milk, because that's where love comes from."

How about their mother? A few days before arriving at my one-year milestone, Linda and I reached our six-year anniversary. We grilled on our deck, used our (rarely used) wedding china, and counted our blessings.

And we talked.

When I first met Linda eleven years ago, she was strong, dynamic, and charismatic. But she was also, in personality, the least dark person I had ever met. Her outlook on life ranged from thumbs-up to thumbs-sideways. By her own admission, she was unsure around the pained emotion, uncertain around the afflicted friend.

This year has changed that. I have watched as Linda absorbed the pummels and emerged not only with her head unbent but with new dimensions in her heart. There were days when her thumb simply had to point down, and the forced practice was transformative.

"My experience makes me want to reach out to people

who are in pain," she said. "Before, I would have been uncomfortable, or unsure of what to say. Now I realize what you say doesn't matter. It's that you say something at all."

Even more, where Linda had always prized self-sufficiency, she now allows—even embraces—her own vulnerability. Particularly for a woman in business, she mentioned, the instinct is to overcompensate, to lead only with strength. But letting people in made her own struggle easier, she said, and in the process made her a more compassionate leader.

Finally, what Linda appreciated about the last year, she said, was that every decision was simpler. It was easier to say No. In the parlance of modern life, the noise was reduced, the signal strengthened. And as she resumes her own stride forward, her wish as a parent, spouse, and friend is to hold on to a fragment of that lucidity.

To keep the clarity.

And you? A few weeks after I was diagnosed, I spoke to a friend who had undergone a similar chemo routine. He lost most of his hearing, the feeling in many of his fingers and toes, and about 15 percent of his cognitive ability. I was horrified.

Today, whatever physical ailments I endure, I am pleased

to report that my mind and spirit are unbowed. My blood may have been ravaged, but my lifeblood remains untouched. I am myself.

But I do have scars—and they flare up at unexpected times.

In April, Linda and I attended the bat mitzvah of a friend's daughter, Alison, at the Boathouse in Central Park. Alison's mother sang a song to her daughter. It was called "Parent's Prayer."

> *May God give you life, and strength, like Joseph's sons. . . .*
> *May God make you like our parents, our blessed ones.*

Like most people in the room, I teared up. But in my case, as my mind turned to our girls and their own life occasions I may miss someday, my tears wouldn't stop. I tried to shield my face but couldn't. I reached for my crutches and fled the room.

Outside, rowboats were in the lake. Families were enjoying the warmest day of the year. The scene was straight out of Manet. For the first time in weeks, I convulsed with tears. And that's when I realized these emotions would never fully disappear. They will reside in my body forever and return at unforeseen moments. The monster within.

During her bat mitzvah ceremony, Alison had read from the Book of Leviticus. While Leviticus is perhaps the least loved book of the Bible, it also contains the Holiness Code, the highest expression of ethics in the Ancient World. One verse, Leviticus 25:10, is quoted on the side of the Liberty Bell: "Proclaim Liberty throughout the land, unto all the inhabitants thereof."

This line refers to a tradition whereby every seven years, farmers are obliged to give their fields a year of rest, a Sabbath. Every seven sets of seven years the land gets an extra year of rest, during which all slaves are to be freed, all families reunited, and all people reminded to uplift the needy and tend the sick. That fiftieth year is called the jubilee year.

And though I'm still shy of fifty, that tradition perfectly captures this past year for me. I was forced to lay fallow. I took off the trappings of contemporary life—vanity, ambition, pretense—and entered into a sort of parallel time where I was compelled to do things the Bible envisions. Be needy. Be a stranger. Be uplifted by those around me. Be reunited with the ones I love.

My Lost Year was my Jubilee Year.

And the jubilation, such as it was, lay exactly where God always knew it would: In lying fallow, I became more fertile. In taking pause, I planted the seeds for a healthier future.

Naturally I worry that I might forget what I learned. I might slip back into the easy tug of whatever vices attract. Having taken off those old clothes, I am tempted to pull them out of my closet and resume my old life as if nothing happened.

But far beneath those clothes I have a lasting reminder of where I've been. In the Book of Genesis, Jacob wrestles with an angel one night and comes to a standstill. The angel leaves a mark on Jacob's thigh to commemorate his struggle. Forever after Jacob walks with a limp.

I, too, have a mark on my thigh, and though mine is far less lofty, it's a permanent sign of the wrestling I've endured. Touch it, and it takes me back to the darkest moments of despair and the brightest moments when others came to uplift us.

A few days after the bat mitzvah, Eden came crying to the side of our bed late one night. Monsters had come into her room and tried to take her stuffed puppy, Do-it. "The best way to get rid of monsters is for us to work together as a family," I said. "Would you like me to sleep with Do-it tonight? That way, when the monsters come, I'll say, 'No, Monster, no!' And they'll go down the stairs, out the door, and leave us alone."

Again we had stumbled into a poignant metaphor for our lives. Monsters came into our home last year. They kept us awake for many months, but we worked together as a family, and, for now at least, they've gone down the stairs, out the door, and left us alone. We still shake occasionally in their wake. We have no guarantees they won't come back. But if they do, we know that the most effective defense we can muster is the best offense we have: to work together as a family.

Thank you for joining our family this year. Thank you to the friend who sent a postcard every day. To the friends and relatives who sent notes, bits of beauty, and casseroles. To those who pushed the swings, repotted the plants, and dried our tears. To those who just read these words, thought for a second, or prayed.

And as this year closes and these letters grow further apart, we turn our thoughts to you. May you find an ounce of jubilation in your own pain, may you enjoin your own fears, "No, Monster, no!," and may you drink from a bottomless glass of milk and remember where love comes from.

And one of these days, please, may you take a walk for me.

Love,

Bruce

23

TAKE A WALK WITH A TURTLE

THE OPENING LINE OF THE tune "Danny by My Side" captures the fantasy. "The Brooklyn Bridge on Sunday is known as lovers' lane." A soldier in *A Tree Grows in Brooklyn* expresses the lure. "I thought if ever I got to New York, I'd like to walk across the Brooklyn Bridge."

It was called "the future of civilization" by its builder, "the grandeur of its age" by a booster. "Babylon had her hanging gardens, Nineveh her towers, Rome her Coliseum," crooned a congressman. "Let us have this great monument to progress."

And for me, in its 126th year, it was the rainbow at the end of my storm.

"Come on, girls," I said one morning. "We're going to take a walk across the Brooklyn Bridge."

"Yippee!" Tybee shouted. "Can we bring a compass?"

"Hooray!" Eden echoed. "Can we have a picnic, too?"

———

TWO HOURS LATER WE were out the door, after one crying fit, four changes of clothes, three lunges of sunscreen, and at least one bellowed threat that there would be no special treats for the rest of their lives. Maybe someone should warn all those lovers on the bridge. Some monuments defy improvement: Four-year-olds are never-changing.

And just when you think you've maxed out on exasperation, they save themselves. As we passed Walt Whitman Park and turned onto the bridge, Tybee looked up at me with her perfect ponytail and said, "Daddy, can you tell us how the bridge was built?"

From the beginning it was shadowed by sorrow and symbolized rebirth. Conceived in the wake of the Civil War, the longest suspension bridge in the world would link the human hive of Manhattan with the backwater of Brooklyn and prove that science could trump human misery. Engineer John Roebling promised one additional feature, the first-ever elevated promenade, which would allow "people of leisure, and old and young invalids, to promenade over the bridge on fine days, in order to enjoy the beautiful views and fine air."

Roebling knew something about misery. An immigrant from Germany, he held séances with his dead wife while designing the bridge and died himself before construction began when a ferry crushed his toes, giving him tetanus. His son, Washington, who took over, came down with a crippling case of the bends while working on the bridge underwater. He was forced to spend the final years of work confined to his home in Brooklyn Heights, unable to read or talk, staring at his masterpiece through an eyepiece. Twenty people died during the decade and a half it took to construct the bridge.

But the bridge also symbolized recovery—for invalids, bereft New Yorkers, and the nation alike. "The shapes arise!" said Brooklyn resident Walt Whitman.

The Brooklyn Bridge embodied for its contemporaries what it became for me: a symbol of affirmation, an arc of renewal.

A parabola of open road.

As we climbed the ramp toward the first tower, we settled into our familial gait. Tybee and Eden flanked Linda, skipping, jumping, and practicing their "rock star" poses, a series of Mick Jagger–like contortions that involved cocking their hips, flipping back their hair, and flinging open their arms, as if to say, "Aren't I fab?" I was bringing up the rear on crutches.

Soon enough our singer-songwriters had made up a tune:

We're walking across the Brooklyn Bridge
Our daddy has stitches and a scar
We're walking across the Brooklyn Bridge
Don't worry, it's not that far!
We're walking across the Brooklyn Bridge
And singing just like a rock star!

Since walking was the first thing I lost when I got sick, I spent much of the months that followed contemplating this most elemental of human acts. Walking upright, or bipedalism, is considered the threshold of being human, the skill that most distinguishes us from our ancestors. It's also immune to improvement. Ever since humans began walking four million years ago, the act has been essentially unchanged. Every step, my physical therapist observed, is a tragedy waiting to happen: You nearly stumble with one leg, then catch yourself with the other. It's a constant struggle against gravity, clumsiness, and misfortune.

But walking can also be the source of meaning. As long as humans have worshiped gods, they have walked to get closer to them. In the Bible, the greatest spiritual breakthroughs occur when the heroes are on journeys: Abraham going forth to the Promised Land; the Israelites crossing the Red Sea; Israel being dispatched to Babylon. From the Haj to the Stations of the Cross, the greatest pilgrimages involve walking. And many pilgrims purposefully make their gait more arduous—with bare feet, awkward clothing, or pebbles in their shoes—in order to slow their pace even more.

Now I understand why.

The simplest consequence of walking on crutches is that you walk slower. Every step must be a necessary one. In my case, the propulsion and pain were distributed throughout my body, from the pinch under my arms to the tingling of my toes. More than bipedal, walking on crutches is full-bodied. Along the way, it makes you more human.

For starters, the act of disrupting your pace brings you into contact with more people. We weren't fifteen steps onto the bridge before a group of men said to me, "Whoa! You're doing this on crutches?! Good luck!" It also creates a bond with others who are slowed, disrupted, or struggling with their own displacement. You develop a citizenship of the estranged. In just the few days before our crossing, I quipped with a businessman in a knee brace, offered to trade maladies with a man in a neck brace, and patted the back of a woman in a walker.

At the risk of admission: I was never nicer than when I was on crutches.

During a visit to New York in the years before the bridge was built, Mark Twain described a desert of solitude, buzzing with impatient hurriers. His portrait captures most people I know today. "Every man seems to feel that he has got the duties of two lifetimes to accomplish in one, and so he rushes, rushes, rushes, and never has time to be companionable—never has any time at his disposal to fool away on matters which do not involve dollars and duty and business."

Few things rupture this tempo more than the inability to hurry. And the interruption becomes an invitation. Stripped of status and authority, the invalid becomes open to community. Going fast, you head only for your destination and inevitably arrive alone. You assert yourself on the world. Going slow, you allow yourself to encounter your surroundings and invariably arrive helped along by strangers.

You discover.

In the 1840s, when walking was just becoming a source of recreation across Europe, a new type of pedestrian appeared in Paris. He was called a flaneur, one who ambled the arcades and strolled the parks in a silent labyrinth of observation and leisure. One emblem of that idleness was the fashion among flaneurs to take a turtle for walks and let the reptile set the pace.

As a paean to slow-moving, I love this notion. And it seems particularly appropriate for the Brooklyn Bridge, which has its own history of Noah-like crossings. The first person to ride across in a carriage took along a rooster; cattle were charged a nickel to cross in those days, sheep and hogs two cents; and soon after the bridge opened, P. T. Barnum herded twenty-one elephants across the main thoroughfare, before deeming it satisfactorily solid.

Above all, I could relate to the flaneur's commitment to the measured tempo. The single most common shard of wisdom I encountered in my excavations of fatherhood—from my grandfather's tapes to my father to my surgeon—was, "Don't be in a hurry." Slow down.

Take a walk with a turtle.

And behold the world in pause.

⸺

AND EVERY ONCE IN a while, stop entirely.

We reached the apex of the bridge. It was just before noon. Eden wanted to eat her picnic immediately, while Tybee was more interested in ogling the joggers wearing no shirts. "Daddy, when are you going to take your shirt off?" she asked. We found a sheltered spot against the face of the tower and spread out bagels, cream cheese, fruit, and milk. A grape rolled through a gap in the planks onto the cars passing beneath us, and Tybee wondered if she could squeeze through and retrieve it. "I think I would have to be very tiny," she said.

"Girls, guess what?" I said. "After lunch, I have a surprise!"

"Oooh, cupcakes?!" Eden cooed.

"No, not something to eat," I said. "Something to do."

Whitman, himself a well-known walker, frequently crossed the river from Brooklyn to Manhattan. His sentiments to those who might cross after him were the same I would speak to my daughters were they to cross someday without me.

> *Just as you feel when you look on the river and*
> *sky, so I felt;*
> *Just as you are refresh'd by the gladness of the*
> *river and the bright flow, I*
> *was refresh'd . . .*
> *These, and all else, were to me the same as they*
> *are to you.*

Above all, I would urge them to cross as often as possible, and be able to say, as Whitman did, "I too *lived*."

When our picnic ended, we packed away the half-eaten bagels and empty grape stems. "I wonder what Daddy's surprise is!?" Linda said. The girls rubbed their hands together. The cyclists and joggers were zooming past us now, blowing whistles to frighten pedestrians from their path. Teenagers were posing for cell phone pictures. An artist hawked charcoal drawings. Saturday noon was rush hour on the Brooklyn Bridge.

I tugged the girls closer and pulled open my shoulder bag. They reached in and lifted out a small red-and-yellow tablecloth, which I spread onto the wooden planks. They reached in again and retrieved four saucers, four cups, a creamer, and a fractured sugar bowl I had glued together the night before. Finally I retrieved the ultimate accessory.

And just after midday, with Lady Liberty to our left

and the Empire State Building to our right, with hundreds of hurriers bustling around us, and for no other reason than we'd reached the end of a long year, we clinked our cups, tilted our kettle, and held a tea party on top of the world.

———

FOR YEARS I SUFFERED from a recurring dream. I would be walking, or climbing, or fleeing something. And I would stall. My legs would turn to mush, or get trapped in some quicksand, or bog down in some existential mud. Then I would wake up—exhausted, panting, and scared.

I never told anybody about my dream. After a while, maybe a decade, I told myself it was probably about ambition, some deep-rooted fear that I might never get to the place I wanted to get.

Then one day, not long before we set out across the Brooklyn Bridge, I realized that I hadn't had the dream since I'd gotten sick. It was a shocking discovery, sort of like losing a relative you didn't exactly love but had grown accustomed to having around. But in my case, the loss was more eerie. As soon as I couldn't walk, I stopped dreaming that I couldn't walk. In the year that I could barely get anywhere, I stopped dreaming that I couldn't get where I wanted to go.

My revelation presented two possibilities. The first is that my body had somehow known all along about the weakness of my legs. Tipped off by some genetic malfunction, my unknowing mind had sent out warning signs that I would someday be stopped short of my dreams.

The other possibility is the more preferable one. I was no longer dissatisfied. Having slowed my pace of life, I was no longer trying to get to a place I wasn't meant to be. The year I couldn't hurry, I stopped trying to hurry someplace else.

Having finally stopped trying to be someplace else, I was finally happy right where I was.

———

WHEN THE TEA PARTY concluded, I asked the girls whether they would like to continue walking across the length of the bridge, then take a taxi home, or retrace our steps and walk home from here. Eden spoke first. "We want to walk all the way across the bridge *aaand* walk back home!" Linda looked at me and winked. "That's our girls!" she said.

·24·

HUG THE MONSTER

September 1

Dear Tybee and Eden,

The last of the sea oats are bending under the weight of
late summer and the afternoon sun is just stretching out
its amber farewell toward the tidal pools on Tybee beach.
Another summer is ending, and with it our time in this
briny paradise, the offbeat island that has always embodied
for your mother and me the fusion of your two names.

As a writer, I've spent my entire adult life composing
words I hoped others might read. I write these words
in the deepest hope that you don't read them for a long,
long time.

But I write them nonetheless, with the emotions so raw, because I want you to hear them from me.

In your second year of life, you first lit upon words. You forged a friendship with letters and language, and that was a pleasure to watch and a marvel to behold. On your second birthday, your mother and I festooned an inflatable alphabet around our home. The letters didn't stick so well; some were drooping by the time we brought you downstairs in your nightgowns; but Eden took one look at the rainbow of *ABC*s and exclaimed, "All the letters came to visit!"

The next year, with ballet and fairies consuming your fancies, we hung pink and purple tutus in similar garlands around the house. "All the tutus came to visit!"

A few weeks later, I went for a routine doctor's appointment. That doctor sent me to another doctor, then another, until I eventually learned that I had a very rare, very aggressive illness that suddenly put my life in peril. I sat on a stoop on a Manhattan street corner, put my face in my palms, and wept. A few hours later I came home and lay down in bed. You immediately came sprinting in after me. You looked in the mirror, clasped your hands together, and started whirling in a circle in a homemade dance, then collapsed to the floor, giddy with joy. My heart collapsed with you.

I thought of all the hugs I might not give to you, all the kisses I might not get. I envisioned the broken hearts I might not mend, the tears I might not blot. I imagined the giggles I might not hear, the songs I might not make up, the doubts I might not assuage. I tallied all the pithy daddyisms I might not impose on you so frequently until you finally snickered and rolled your eyes. *Try something new every day. Start with the facts, the decisions will make themselves. When all else fails, read the instructions.*

I thought of my voice, and what your life might be like without it.

Three days later I awoke before dawn with an idea of how I might help give you that voice. I would reach out to six men, from all passages in my life, and ask them to be present through the passages in yours. They might whisper to you, sing to you, profess to you, or write to you. They might take you for a ride on a tractor, or take you out back for a talking-to. They might lend you a hand, lift up your chin, or let down your hair. They might simply listen to you.

They would be a swirl of voices I would hang in your life for all time.

"All the daddies came to visit."

And I would call this group of men "The Council of Dads."

The men in this circle aren't my only friends. They're not my only mentors, teachers, or guides. They're not my brother, my sister, or my family. They aren't your daddy, I'm afraid.

But they do constitute various sides of me. They are a narrative of my selves.

In the event of my death, they can carry on my life. If I go silent, they can continue to speak for me.

How you use this Council is up to you. You might ask them about me—what I would have been thinking, what I might have said. You might ask them about you—how you make a tricky decision, how you make a dream come true. You might ask them about themselves.

When I invited each of them to join your Council, I sought from each the single lesson that he might bequeath to you now. Their wisdom, assembled, reads like a psalmbook of living.

Approach the cow
Pack your flip-flops
Don't see the wall
Tend your tadpoles
Live the questions
Harvest miracles

You may understand some of these ideas when you first
hear them; others perhaps you may not understand for
some time. But they are truths as deep as I know. And
I have gathered them, along with like-minded thoughts
from my father, my two grandfathers, and various father
figures in my life, as well as a few from myself I couldn't
resist tossing in (*Always learn to juggle on the side of a hill; Take a
walk with a turtle*), into a handbook of fatherly guidance.

When assembling this counsel I have been reminded
of the great paradox of parenting: Even as we come
to feel we can't live without you, our primary job is to
prepare you to live without us. Our task, in a sense, is to
make ourselves obsolete. As babies, you arrive entirely
dependent; we then spend the coming decades trying to
make you independent, so you can thrive on your own,
without us.

You may face this situation sooner than most, I fear. You
will have your mommy, and she, as you surely know, is a
Council unto herself. Listen to her and you'll learn truths
far deeper than any roomful of men will ever know.

But you might not have your daddy. And where I would
have been in your life, a hole will likely be. You may fill
that hole over the years with love or grief, with anger or
fear, with lollipops or monsters.

All of those are okay.

But whatever you fill the emptiness with, be gentle on yourself. This situation is not your fault. This plight is not your destiny.

The most daring pilots in the world have a motto for how they handle life's greatest tests. The air force teaches its novices that when they face a life-defining challenge, they should not run from their fear. They should embrace it. "Hug the monster," they say. Wrap your arms around your fear, wrestle it into submission, redirect it into a source of resilience and purpose.

Hug the monster, girls.

I can be your arms. Because if you know nothing else about me, know that your daddy loved you. I loved when you climbed on my tummy in the morning and told me that snuggling with Daddy was your favorite time of day. I loved when you snickered at my teasing and groaned at my puns. I loved when you made up songs, played rhyming dictionary, or danced. I especially loved when you curtsied. I even loved when I put you in the crying chair, or raised my voice, or counted "One . . . two . . . two and a *haaalffff . . .*"

I loved when I made a big production out of refusing to

read to you, or get you a stapler, or give you a snack after school, until you gave me a proper hug and kiss. I loved when you reached for my crutches, when you patted my scar. I loved when you looked frightened in my direction, and when you grabbed my finger during fireworks, after I said, "Squeeze me if you're scared."

You can still do that when I'm gone, you know. Just squeeze your fingers together. I'll feel it wherever I am.

A few weeks after you were born, we held a party to introduce you to our friends. I gave a short toast that night. My closing wish was, "May your first word be *adventure* and your last word *love*." I can report that the first half of that wish came true. *Adventure* was one of the first words you learned and one of the words you loved most during those years. Your little lips would curl around its syllables, capturing all the complexity, wonder, and unknown in its meaning.

"We're going on a special adventure," we would say, and your eyes would fill with anticipation.

The second half of that wish—"May your last word be *love*"—is up to you. And if I've learned anything from my illness, it's that we never know when our last word may come. So I beg of you: Be awash in love every day. That love may come from a friend, a relative, a lover, a child.

It may come from all of these, or just one. But if I could leave you with one last bequest: May it always come from each other. Whatever else happens, always comfort your sister.

If nothing else, through each other, you'll always have a connection to your mother and me.

Because if the paradox of being a parent is that we must make ourselves unneeded, the paradox of being a child is that you discover how much you need your parents only after you think you don't. You spend your whole lives making yourself independent. You go forth on your own. And at exactly the moment you stop listening to us, you finally hear what we've been saying all along.

Until then, I'll be waiting. Even if you can't hear me, I'll be whispering in your ear. Even if you can't feel me, I'll be gently pushing you on your own. And even if you can't see me, I'll be holding up my finger for you to squeeze when the monster needs hugging.

Take trips, girls. Take chances. Take off.

And every once in a while, take a walk for me.

Love,
Daddy

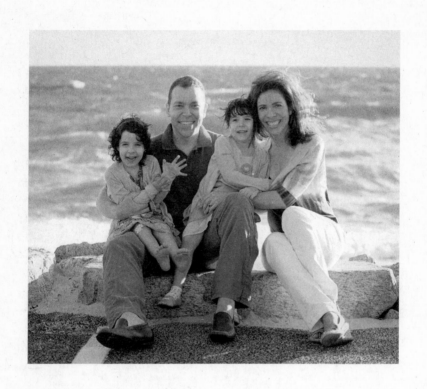

THE COUNCIL CONVENES

THE MEN SCHEMED WITH LINDA. They planned it themselves. And on a sunny Saturday morning in mid-April, they walked through our door in Brooklyn, each bearing a present for Eden and Tybee's fifth birthday. Jeff brought two toy tractors. David carried matching pink softballs, bats, and gloves. No wonder the girls liked having these men in their lives. They scored! We all gathered around the table, and Linda brought out a cake with five candles. And that's when it hit me.

The Council of Dads was in our living room. They had convened for the very first time.

"They're here," Linda whispered in my ear. "And you are, too."

Nearly two years had passed since my diagnosis and

that horrendous first week when I decided to ask these men to be present in the lives of our daughters. I was cancer free now. My leg was steadily regaining mobility. After a year and a half on crutches and nearly nine months on a cane, I was ready to step gingerly into the future. Though my regular follow-ups, quarterly scans, and physical therapy would continue, my energy, spirit, and self had returned. As Dr. Healey said to me, "This is what I hoped for and envisioned when we set out on this journey."

The Council of Dads was a far richer experience than we could have hoped for. That afternoon in our living room, the men sat around and got to know one another. Ben leaned against the banister; Max read the girls a story; Joshua put on the pink softball gloves and chased the girls in the backyard. The men argued about politics, parenting, and height. They teased me mercilessly. The conversation was part locker room, part roast, part support group. Looking at all our middle-age selves at one point, I thought I should have called the group the Council of Bald Spots. After overhearing some of the banter, Linda chimed in: "I always wondered what you guys would talk about. Now I know: midlife crises and sports cars! You're such men!"

As for the girls, they didn't care. They were delighted as they moved from dad to dad, reveling in the private bond they share with each one. They even had nicknames for each of the men: Tractor Jeff because he drives them around on a tractor, Tadpole Ben because he takes them fishing when they go to Savannah, Chocolate-chip David because he bakes cookies with them. Mostly they knew that these men are not just Daddy's friends. They are *their* friends.

That feeling was the most unexpected side effect of the Council. It built a bridge between my friends and my family. Something in our society, I have come to believe, conspires against friendship, especially for busy parents. We have our work; we have our children; but our friends keep getting pushed aside. The Council of Dads proved to be a powerful way to invite our friends into the heart of what's most important in our lives: our kids. Even more, by giving each dad a specific role to play—Travel Dad (Jeff), Values Dad (Max), Dream Dad (David)—serving on the Council avoided becoming a burden. The men like their roles because it allows them to focus on what they're naturally good at; the girls like it because they have something special with each man. (When Joshua came over at Halloween and snuck the girls chocolate bars after we brushed their teeth, I realized that he would be Irresponsibility Dad.)

The girls' warm reaction to having these men in their lives provided the answer to one of the common (and, to me, surprising) questions I got about The Council of Dads. Will you ever disband it? Never. If anything, I can't believe I was a parent for three years without one, and I will certainly never parent without one again. One of the unspoken secrets of parenting, in my experience, is that it can be very lonely—especially for dads, who feel the need to be the Answer Man, Mr. Fix It, the Know-It-All. Maybe our fathers played this role for us, or maybe we interpreted their silence, or awkwardness, to be the mark of their being in total control. For whatever reason, dads today like to think we have all the answers, when often we don't. But now, when I face some tricky question or awkward situation,

I can reach out to these men. Creating a Council of Dads turned fatherhood from a solo sport into a team sport.

And when this book was published days after that gathering, and our story began making its way into the world, I heard the most moving stories from other parents. So many others wanted something similar in their lives. Parents who were ill, worked in dangerous jobs, traveled frequently, or were facing their own mortality suddenly started their own Councils with memberships ranging from three to thirteen. Single parents wanted a Council of Moms or Dads to help them through difficult times. Parents of teenagers wanted Councils because their children were starting to withdraw and need trusted adults who were not their relatives. The United States military started a special program for servicemen and -women to form Councils. Adoptive parents, deeply religious parents, those parents whose kids have interests they can't mentor them on, all found inspiration in this idea. Even grown-ups who had lost their parents started Councils of Moms or Dads to connect retroactively with their own pasts. The response became so overwhelming that I started a website, www.councilofdads.com, where people could share their own stories, download a starter kit with tips for forming their own Councils, and communicate with others who are doing the same thing.

The day The Council of Dads first met, we all had dinner together. Everyone went around the table and spoke of how the experience had changed him. Linda spoke, too, about how these men had become her support group also. One of the men felt the Council helped replace the voice of his *own* father. Another took the advice he gave our girls and changed how he parents his own children. The last person to speak was Ben Sherwood. I call him Question Dad. He calls himself The Contrarian.

"When I first heard the idea of the Council, I rejected it," he said. "You would triumph over your illness. We wouldn't need to exist. Today I realized I was wrong. Whether we're healthy or sick, male or female, we all need to be surrounded by the ones we love. And seeing the looks on the girls' faces today, I now know we all need our own Council."

That night I discovered the most enduring impact of The Council of Dads. Linda and I did it for our girls.

But it really changed all of us.

SAY PLEASE AND THANK YOU

An enormous team of people contributed to saving my life.

Dr. Diana Santini gave me the alkaline phosphatase test that launched me on this journey, then pushed me to get the follow-up tests. Dr. Beth Shubin-Stein took over my case and provided invaluable advice and introductions. Dr. John Healey is the most inspiring doctor I know and one of the most compelling people I've ever met. Dr. Robert Maki was extraordinarily generous with advice, acumen, and fellowship through some very dark and difficult months. Dr. Bebak Mehrara is a gentleman and a master surgeon. Dr. Alison Haimes was a daily font of wisdom and advice, and she became an intimate member of our family through her constant presence during this ordeal.

A warm appreciation to the many teams of medical professionals who answered our calls, calmed our nerves, and held our hands. In Dr. Healey's office: Jodi Roth, Matthew Steensma, and Fazel Khan. In Dr. Maki's office: Stephen Layne, Linda Ahn, Elizabeth Rodriguez. In the fifth-floor chemo clinic: Sarah Duncan, Stacy O'Neill, Sara Martinez, Ray Rodriguez, Heather Goettsch, and Karen Gormsmen, among others.

For key support along the way, thank you to Dr. Joe Bender, Dr. Bob Mayer, Dr. Alan Muney, and David Davidoff. And a rousing deep knee bend and short jig on the dance floor to the incomparably sharp Theresa Chiaia and her entire team at the Sports Rehabilitation Department at the Hospital for Special Surgery.

I was deeply touched and comforted by the extraordinary goodness of Clarissa and Edgar Bronfman Jr. We were equally overwhelmed by the compassion of Belle and Wences Casares, Melissa and Tim Draper, Paul Fribourg, Ann and Jason Green, Amy and John Griffin, and Peter Kellner.

To all the friends and family around the world who sent expressions of love; poems, prayers, and paisley afghans; and dishes for our casserole club.

To those who offered just the right support at just the right time: Jeanne Ackman, Karen and Bill Ackman, Sunny Bates, Nick Beim, Kimberly Braswell, Justin Castillo, Andy Cowan, Tracey and David Frankel, Caterina Fake, Jan and Gordon Franz, Avner Goren, Diane Galligan and Brendan Hasenstab, Wes Gardenswartz, Lisa Kapp, David Kramer, Corby Kummer, Jane Lear, Lia Levenson and Evan Oppenheimer, Susan Levy, Serge Lippe, Ilene Leff, Andrea Mail, Becca and Dickie Plofker, Joanna Rees and John Hamm, Gretchen Rubin, Peter Schuck, Daniel Schwartz, Chip Seelig, David Shenk, Ken Shubin Stein, Joe Weisberg, Alexi Worth, and Judy and Bob Wunsch.

To those who saw the pain up close and kept coming back: Laura Benjamin, Karen Lehrman Bloch and Bradley Bloch, Susan Chumsky, Karen Essex, Lauren Schneider, and Teresa Tritch.

To those who share the journey: Raul Buelvas, Olivia Fox, and Todd Haimes.

Special thanks to Megan Brown, Karen Glimmerveen, Tim Hawkins, Soribel Holguin, Jazie Ingram, and Greg Takoudes.

I am grateful for the many people I work with who drew closer to us during this time: Alan Berger, Helen Churko, Susan Ellingwood, Craig Jacobson, Lynn Goldberg, Beth Middleworth, Brian Pike, Lucy Lepage and Carlton Sedgeley, Roger Triemstra, and Sally Willcox.

My friends and colleagues at HarperCollins expressed extraordinary commitment at the outset of this experience, and nearly every day along the way. I am forever appreciative of Brian Murray, Michael Morrison, and Liate Stehlik for their continued presence and support. Seale Ballenger, Lynn Grady, Tavia Kowalchuk, Shawn Nicholls, Sharyn Rosenblum, Mary Schuck, Danny Goldstein, and Nicole Chismar are treasured colleagues. In twenty years of writing books, I have never worked more closely or had a more trusted and valued partnership with an editor than I have with Henry Ferris.

A special hug for Lisa Gallagher, who believed from the very beginning.

All the Feilers and Rottenbergs were always within earshot and arm's length, and willing to leave their own lives behind to help us cope with ours. I can only hope that the splatters of misery I sometimes spread along the way did not conceal the love I so profoundly experienced.

The six men who appear in this book help form the backbone of my life. In addition to the steady pulse of friendship they shared throughout this journey, they all welcomed my probing eye into the deepest secrets of their lives and allowed me to mine them for my girls. I vow in however many days I have left to try to reach to the standards of humanity, joy, and compassion they already embody for me and my children.

Linda Rottenberg is the beating heart that informs every word in these pages. She managed during this unimaginable ordeal to conceal her own fear just enough to allow herself to wipe away some of mine. I love discovering nearly every day the magical parts of her being that emerge in our daughters. And I am profoundly comforted that should my Council of Dads ever need to convene for its original purpose, she will guide them with her effortless grace.

Tybee and Eden: This book is for you. I dread the day you will read it, but I trust you know it's true. And I hope that you will always remember the words I would sing to you before you went to sleep—"Daddy-Daddy loves you very, very . . . " and the word you would whisper back: "Much."

For tips on creating your own Council of Dads or Council of Moms, to share your story and keep the conversation going, or to help find a cure for sarcomas and other rare cancers, please visit brucefeiler.com or councilofdads.com.

BOOKS BY BRUCE FEILER

AMERICA'S PROPHET
ISBN 978-0-06-172627-9 (paperback)
"This is one of the most original, intelligent, and endlessly fascinating books I have read in years." —Simon Winchester

WHERE GOD WAS BORN
A Daring Adventure Through the Bible's Greatest Stories
ISBN 978-0-06-057489-5 (paperback)
"Another absorbing blend of travelogue, history, Bible commentary, memoir, current events, and passionate preaching." —*Publishers Weekly*

WALKING THE BIBLE
A Journey by Land Through the Five Books of Moses
ISBN 978-0-06-083863-8 (paperback)
"An instant classic." —*Washington Post Book World*

WALKING THE BIBLE
A Photographic Journey
ISBN 978-0-06-079904-5 (hardcover)
The companion to the PBS series based on Feiler's bestseller.

ABRAHAM
A Journey to the Heart of Three Faiths
ISBN 978-0-06-083866-9 (paperback)
"A winning mix of insight, passion, and historical research." —*Christian Science Monitor*

LEARNING TO BOW
Inside the Heart of Japan
ISBN 978-0-06-057720-9 (paperback)
"A refreshingly original look at Japan." —*Atlanta Journal-Constitution*

LOOKING FOR CLASS
Days and Nights at Oxford and Cambridge
ISBN 978-0-06-052703-7 (paperback)
"Full of companionable characters, solid information, and wit." —Scott Turow

UNDER THE BIG TOP
A Season with the Circus
ISBN 978-0-06-052702-0 (paperback)
"A colorful, sometimes unsettling pageant of circus life." —*Entertainment Weekly*

Visit www.BruceFeiler.com and www.AuthorTracker.com
for exclusive information on your favorite HarperCollins authors.

Available wherever books are sold, or call 1-800-331-3761 to order.